The Healer's Calling

The Healer's Calling

Women and Medicine in Early New England

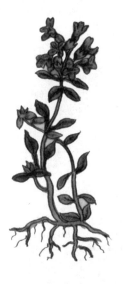

Rebecca J. Tannenbaum

CORNELL UNIVERSITY PRESS
Ithaca and London

First published 2002 by Cornell University Press

Printed in the United States of America

Library of Congress Cataloging-in-Publication Data

Tannenbaum, Rebecca J. (Rebecca Jo)
    The healer's calling : women and medicine in early New England /
Rebecca J. Tannenbaum.
        p. cm.
Includes bibliographical references and index.
    ISBN 0-8014-3826-8
    1. Women in medicine—New England—History—17th century.   2. Women in medicine—New England—History—18th century.   3. New England—History—Colonial period, ca. 1600-1775.   I. Title.
    R692 .T364 2002   2001007137

Cornell University Press strives to use environmentally responsible suppliers and materials to the fullest extent possible in the publishing of its books. Such materials include vegetable-based, low-VOC inks and acid-free papers that are recycled, totally chlorine-free, or partly composed of nonwood fibers. For further information, visit our website at www.cornellpress.cornell.edu.

Cloth printing   10 9 8 7 6 5 4 3 2 1

In memory of my grandmother
Jane Swope Angle
and her grandmother
Sadie Traxler Swope

Strength and honor are her clothing;
and she shall rejoice in time to come.

PROVERBS 31:25

Contents

PART II: AUTHORITY

[5]
CALLED TO COURT
Women Healers as Witnesses and Authorities
93

[6]
CALLING THE DOCTORESS
Commercial Practice
114

EPILOGUE
The Changing Context of the Healer's Calling
135

NOTES
153

INDEX
173

Preface

THE WRITING OF HISTORY, like many other kinds of writing, depends on a series of images. These historical images, accurate or not, have great persistence. Teachers and writers of history have a responsibility to revise and complicate old images with new facts and new interpretations. With this book, I hope to transform the image of life in early New England with a study of women medical practitioners and their relationships with their families, their communities, and their male counterparts. Tracing these relationships has made it apparent that medical practice enabled women to participate in the world beyond the household and allowed them to exercise surprising autonomy and authority.

One popular image of the early New England housewife might show a woman bending over a hearth, stirring the contents of a bubbling pot, surrounded by her children. Another image might picture her sitting in her assigned pew at the local meetinghouse. There is certainly truth in these portrayals—women were efficient household managers and more pious than their male kin. However, these images are incomplete. While the ideal New England woman was supposed to be meek and submissive, the reality was quite different. Women seized as many opportunities as they could to claim authority and assert their own interests. Medical practice was one important way they did so.

I also hope my study of women healers will transform the image of early American medicine. An image of the early American doctor that parallels that of the housewife might portray a somber man of good family who carries an instrument case full of lancets and strong purgative drugs. He speaks learnedly of Hippocrates and Galen, and perhaps also of Paracelsus and Harvey. However, as this study makes clear, learned physicians were in the minority, even among male practitioners, and at least in British North America, the "medical man" might just as likely have been a woman.

Even the terms "medicine" and "medical practice" are transformed when women healers enter the picture. When twenty-first-century readers see these words, they conjure up an image quite different from the seventeenth-century reality. At that time, medicine was not a matter for highly educated, licensed professionals who had a distinct personal and social identity as physicians. Nor was it an arcane body of knowledge accessible only to those professionals. Definitions of medicine were more fluid and included the herbal remedies of a village housewife as well as the elaborate, chemically based drugs of a university-educated physician. Indeed, in some ways it is inappropriate to use words like *medicine* and *medical practice* to describe how the sick were cared for in the early modern world. The people of the time would have used words like *physick, healing,* and *midwifery* to describe what they were doing. In the seventeenth century, the healing methods closest to the modern definition of medicine were what might be called elite practice: that of university-educated "gentlemen" who were licensed by the Royal College of Physicians. This definition covers only a small minority of those who practiced physick or healing.

However, if we define medicine in a different way, it is an appropriate word. If medicine is a system of caring for the sick that includes diagnosis, the making of medicines, and physical support and manipulation of the patient, then what most seventeenth-century practitioners did was indeed practice medicine. And if we define anyone who performs these acts as a medical practitioner, then most seventeenth-century women were medical practitioners.

Finding documentation on women practitioners—or any type of healer—in early American sources can be a daunting task. There are a few treasures lurking in the archives, such as a medicinal recipe book kept by four generations of women in Marlborough, Massachusetts. However, for the most part, a researcher is left with the usual group of documents available to social historians: depositions taken for county courts; diaries, letters, and account books (written, for the most part, by men); and an assortment of published material, ranging from almanacs to gardening manuals to household advice books.

The advantage of using these "indirect" sources is that they demonstrate the ways in which healing was an inherent part of everyday life, and illustrate the participation of healers in almost every event.

The ubiquity of women healers suggests that healing had important social meanings, but it takes some close examination to find those meanings in the sources. If we look closely at two ordinary scenes where women practiced medicine, we can begin to see what healing meant to the women who practiced it.

Samuel Sewall recorded the first scene in his diary in January of 1702. At dawn on January 2, he went to fetch women—three neighbors and a midwife—to attend his wife in labor. While he was out, he stopped at the home of the minister, Mr. Willard, to ask him to "call on God" on Mrs. Sewall's behalf. When Mr. Sewall returned home, the women asked him to join them for a prayer. Sewall then withdrew. He spent the morning in another room while the women conducted the birth. After the Sewalls' daughter was born, Mr. Sewall engaged a wet nurse to take charge of the infant and to sit with his convalescent wife while she recovered. Despite the nurse's vigilance, complications arose. Mrs. Sewall developed a fever and became "something delirious." Mr. Sewall had to spring into action once more to fetch another healer—this time a male physician, Dr. Oakes. Luckily, the fever did not linger, and Mrs. Sewall recovered—so well, in fact, that she was able to host a dinner party for her female birth attendants two weeks later.[1]

Running through this scene are tendrils and threads of different communities. First and foremost was the community of women found in every birthing room and around almost every sickbed. The female attendants were a medical necessity during childbirth. In addition, the long hours of intimate watching and waiting created relationships that did not disappear when the child was born. The women lingered after the birth to take care of the new mother and the infant. Once she was well enough to get out of bed, Mrs. Sewall acknowledged her attendants' importance by serving them an elaborate dinner including treats such as turkey pie, roast beef, and tarts. These communities of women had important functions in women's everyday lives as well, even when they were not pregnant, nursing, or ill. Women's medical networks bound families and communities together, served as a public forum where women could voice their concerns and complaints, and became a base from which some women could mount campaigns to address social and political issues.

Samuel Sewall was also part of this community. He was the one who brought the women together. He participated in at least one childbirth ritual when he prayed with his wife and her attendants. Before he even returned home from his errands, however, he performed a male childbirth ritual of his own: he went to the minister and asked him to pray for his wife. Through her husband, Mrs. Sewall was linked to the community of high-ranking men to which her husband belonged. That community also had a stake in her welfare. Finally, Sewall linked his family to yet another part of the community when he called a male physician to see to his wife's fever, linking the midwife and the wet nurse to the physician. Women's communities were always linked to men's. This linkage meant that events taking place within the single-sex gatherings in birthing rooms had resonance for all the inhabitants of a town.

A second scene reveals a different theme. Here, we are given a glimpse inside another birthing room. This time it is not the well-appointed chamber of Mrs. Sewall but the pallet bed of an unmarried servant named Hannah Adams. Despite her circumstances, Adams was still surrounded by a group of community women—and it is one of those women who described the scene. Anne Thurley gave a deposition before Commissioner Joseph Woodbridge of the Essex County Court in Massachusetts concerning the father of Adams's illegitimate child. The midwife, Goodwife Dole, had asked Adams several times who the father was, including at the "extremity of her pain." Each time, Adams repeated the same name, Joseph Mayo. "Come life, come death," Thurley testified, "she must say it was his." The last time she was asked, Adams "wept when she so spake." Such repeated assertions convinced the attendants that Adams was telling the truth, despite Mayo's equally adamant denials. Now, Thurley and another woman, Constance Moores, had come to court to testify to what they witnessed, and to ensure that the child would be supported by Mayo rather than becoming a public charge.[2]

Community plays a part here too: the childbed gathering, the concern for public morals, and the town's finances. But another element also arises: the public authority of women healers. The midwife, in particular, is a powerful figure. Goodwife Dole performed the "examination" of Adams while she was in labor. Dole was not lax in her enforcement of the community norm; she interrogated Adams over and over again, despite Adams's "sharp and hard" labor. Dole did not relent until Adams was in tears—from pain, fear, and frustration at not being taken at her word. A woman healer's authority began with her power over other women.

A midwife's power extended beyond the birth chamber. It was her duty to name the child's father before the court. When a midwife did so, provided that her examination had been vigorous enough, her word was believed, even if the man named denied the charge. In the case of Hannah Adams, Dole was unable to attend the court hearing. The other women who had been at Adams's labor performed this duty in Dole's stead. When they did so, they too partook of the midwife's legal authority. Joseph Mayo and other men like him were thus at the mercy of women healers. In these circumstances, women could coerce men into acts they were reluctant to perform, such as paying to support their illegitimate children.

Community ties and positions of authority were the two main results of women's medical practice. Women used their healing skills to gain advantages for themselves, their families, and their community factions. In all cases, the consequences of their behavior had a double edge. Under some circumstances, healing could be empowering for both the healer and other women. In others, women healers turned against their patients, such as when they chose to testify against them. In still others, women healers found that their practices brought serious social and legal consequences down on their heads.

Any discussion of social and legal sanctions for women inevitably leads to another image of the early New England woman: the witch. In many ways the image of the witch counters that of the housewife. The witch is sharp-tongued, widowed, and childless. The pot on her hearth does not contain porridge but a poison or a love potion—or a medicine. Witchcraft and healing were linked in the seventeenth century, in the same way that they are in popular images of colonial women today. However, that linkage is more complex than it first appears. The majority of women healers practiced completely free of all social sanction, including witchcraft accusations. Others fell under suspicion but were never formally accused or were acquitted at their trials. A small minority were convicted and executed. What made the difference? It was not the practice of medicine itself that caused some women to become suspect, but the way they practiced it. A careful examination of which healers were accused and under what circumstances demonstrates the delicate balance between self-assertion and feminine meekness that early American women negotiated on a daily basis.

This book explores the many ways these themes—community, authority, and the extent and limits of women's power—played out in early New England towns and farms. Part 1 looks at the theme of community. Chapter 1 begins with a description of healing in the seventeenth century: concepts of health and disease, theories of medicine, and the types of medical practitioners available. It then describes the hierarchies of gender, social rank, and education that distinguished different types of healers, and discusses how these hierarchies affected the relationship between female healers and their male counterparts. From this big picture, the book moves on to describe healing in the smallest of communities: the household. Chapter 2 describes housewives' domestic medicine, which included techniques ranging from herbal medicines and nursing care to abortion and healing magic.

The second half of part 1 discusses two different ways in which healers and healing interacted with ideas of community. As we saw in the two vignettes presented earlier, women formed social networks that coalesced around sickbeds and childbirths. Chapter 3 describes the origins, structure, and function of these medical networks, the ways women manipulated them to their own advantage, and the ways in which male social networks intersected with the women's medical community. The connections between women healers and the wider society went beyond the sickroom. Chapter 4 discusses the ways social rank and gender interacted in the practice of medicine. It focuses on two case studies of high-ranking women healers. The first is about the relationship between the healer Elizabeth Davenport, a minister's wife in New Haven Colony, and John Winthrop Jr., governor of Connecticut and practicing physician. Their relationship served to uphold existing social hierarchies, teaching their mutual patients respect for their betters. At the same time, Davenport and Winthrop never forgot the hierarchies of gender, which ensured that Davenport always deferred to Winthrop in medical matters. The second case study is a marked contrast to the first. It focuses on the healer, midwife, and religious dissident Ann Hutchinson, who used her medical skills not to support the status quo, as Elizabeth Davenport did, but to mount a challenge to the religious and political power structure.

Part 2 takes up the theme of authority—both its uses and its limits. Midwives and other women healers were frequent witnesses in court proceedings. Chapter 5 explores their legal authority and the considerable autonomy they had in gathering and presenting evidence in the masculine public arena. Because of this authority, women healers were objects of both respect and fear in their communities, and because of their autonomy, they had to make choices about how best to use their power. The next chapter looks at another group of women who shared this autonomy and authority. Some women were able to make their living practicing medicine, and they competed directly with male physicians for patients. Such independent "doctoresses" were vulnerable to lawsuits and witchcraft accusations. This chapter includes a close analysis of some court proceedings. The court cases demonstrate the independence of these practitioners, the consequences for stretching that authority too far, and male physicians' reactions to the competition these women represented.

Changes in medicine and gender ideologies brought changes in the role of women healers. The book ends with an epilogue that briefly traces these changes through the early nineteenth century. As the eighteenth century wore on, educated male physicians became more available to patients, and women's traditional knowledge and lay practices became devalued, even as patients continued to use women healers. One section of the epilogue follows the medical choices of one family over the course of the eighteenth century. This family, like many others, began to use male doctors in conjunction with female practitioners. However, women's practice never died out. Midwives, in particular, continued to practice. By the early nineteenth century, women began to agitate for admission to medical schools, and some became successful "physicians" even after they were denied a degree. The final pages discuss the career of Elizabeth Blackwell, the first American woman to be admitted to medical school.

The title of this work plays on a familiar term from Puritan theology and social life: the calling. There were two kinds of calling. One was general and required all people to serve and worship God. The second concerned an individual's life course and vocation. An individual's calling was a way of doing his or her part in working out God's higher plan. Some young men agonized over a choice of a calling, trying to decipher what God's will and plan was for them. Some of these young men heard the call to medical practice—either as a gentleman physician, a military surgeon, or an itinerant doctor. Healing the sick was profitable work and a way of serving both God and the community.[3]

Women had fewer choices of callings. Their first call was to take care of their households. However, medical care was an inherent part of that work. Housewives raised medicinal plants, sat up all night with sick children, and made medicines for their families. Medicine was part of a religious call as well. For the pious, healing one's neighbors was an occasion for charity and service to others and God. It was also a chance to act as a moral enforcer: the gossip exchanged at sickbeds and at childbirth gatherings was a chance to discuss the behavior of neighbors and perhaps reprimand those who had overstepped the bounds of propriety. If such measures failed, midwives and other healers often had the chance to send wrongdoers to court for further action.

Healing entered into all the roles of the virtuous woman—as a household manager, as a Christian, as a concerned neighbor. Indeed, adding healing to the picture transforms our image of the colonial goodwife. When we imagine her stirring a pot on the hearth, we need to also see her distilling a medicine. When we see her instructing her children in proper conduct, we need to also see her binding up their cuts and setting their broken bones. When we describe her as a pious Christian, we need to see her taking medicines to the bedside of a poor, sick neighbor. When we imagine her as a submissive wife, we need to see her giving testimony in court that brings consequences to bear on male fornicators and rapists. Women provided a large part of the medical care in early colonial New England, a practice that tied them to all parts of their communities and gave them access to social and legal authority.

Many individuals and institutions have contributed to this book. Financial support is crucial to any intellectual enterprise, and several institutions have helped smooth the way for this project. A Kate B. and Hall J. Peterson fellowship at the American Antiquarian Society (AAS) supported a crucial month of research at the AAS. A Yale University dissertation fellowship supported me for a year while I wrote the first draft; a sabbatical leave from the University of Illinois at Chicago allowed me to finish the final version.

The most important intellectual support came from three people: John Demos, Nancy Cott, and John Harley Warner. John Demos, in particular, has been with this work from the beginning. As a mentor, he opened the door to the past in ways I had never expected. I am particularly grateful for his confidence in me and my project. John Warner and Nancy Cott also contributed their expertise. Nancy Cott was especially good at giving me straight talk about the strengths and weaknesses of my argument, and at keeping my historiographic references current. In addition to sharing his seemingly inexhaustible knowledge of the history of medicine, John Warner never let me get by with a fuzzy definition or an imprecise term. I am deeply indebted to all three for their support, their criticisms, and their dedication to history.

Others also gave time and thought to supporting this project. The staff at the AAS were extremely helpful and pointed me toward several important sources. During my stay at the AAS, I met Ross Beales, who graciously shared with me some of his computer analyses of the Ebenezer Parkman diary. Edward Jurkowitz suggested a book to me that clarified my thinking for chapter 1. The undergraduate students in my history of medicine class at the University of Illinois at Chicago inspired me with their enthusiasm for the project. I also have benefited from the critical eyes of several people who read and commented on drafts of chapters: Bernard Bailyn, Beatrix Hoffman, Jane Kamensky, Jill Lepore, Clare Lyons, Shirley Tannenbaum, and the members of the Newberry Seminar on Early American History. Finally, I must thank several people at Cornell University Press. Peter Agree was the first to see the potential in this project, and Sheri Englund saw it through to completion. The anonymous readers for the press gave me a set of comments that were essential in giving the book its final shape.

My husband, Charles Bailyn, has contributed in every way imaginable. He has read more drafts of this book than I care to admit (or than he cares to remember). He deserves more thanks than I can give him here. And of course, no set of acknowledgments would be complete without mentioning our dog Pippin, a small but indomitable force for good.

This book is dedicated to two remarkable women. My maternal grandmother, Jane Swope Angle, died while I was still researching this book, and thus never had a chance to read it. Even so, I think she would recognize herself in some of the women portrayed in its pages. Like a colonial goodwife, she valued good housewifery, community service, and the importance of using the resources at hand to fight necessary battles. I never knew my great-great-grandmother Sadie

Traxler Swope, but she was a regular character in family stories. Like her granddaughter Jane Swope, she was a pillar of the community and of her church, and may have been what her colonial forebears called a "cunning woman." She made herbal medicines, knew how to charm away warts and predict marriages, and laid out the dead for burial. She also tried her hand at politics—she was the first woman to run for public office in Franklin County, Pennsylvania. I am proud to be descended from these women and am particularly proud to dedicate this book to their memory.

PART 1: *Community*

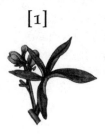

Calling the Healers

Early Modern Medicine and Colonial Practitioners

MARY BRIGHAM WAS IN A quandary. Her husband had a chronic rash that covered his hands with weeping sores and blisters. Her usual remedy had not brought any relief. Eager for another medicine to try, she found a recipe in her family notebook. This one had come from a male doctor, and she thought it might work better than the salves and poultices her female neighbors had suggested. She followed the directions carefully, boiling a variety of herbs with spring water and wine, soaking woolen cloths in the liquid, and wrapping them around her husband's hands.[1]

Medicine was not the exclusive domain of elite professionals in British North America. In seventeenth-century England and its colonies, domestic medicine did not differ much from learned medicine. Both practitioners and patients used the same language to discuss healing and disease, and both groups understood illness in the same way. In the American colonies, this situation was amplified by the scarcity of elite practitioners. In this context, women healers were ubiquitous—at sickbeds, at childbirths, and in the community. These female practitioners practiced their craft in the company of male colleagues, with whom they developed a variety of hierarchical relationships.[2]

EARLY MODERN MEDICINE

Historians of medicine have often characterized the seventeenth century as the time when medicine began to become recognizably "scientific." In England, William Harvey published his 1628 treatise describing the circulation of the blood. Thomas Sydenham was beginning to move away from the teachings of the ancients and develop his own theories of the classification and etiology of disease. The Swiss chemist Paracelsus did similar work, changing the traditional reliance on herbal medicines to a system based on chemical principles.[3]

Some of this medical theory crossed the ocean to the colonies. A few early New England intellectuals, such as Increase and Cotton Mather, followed European scientific ideas and promulgated them in America. Others, such as Governor John Winthrop Jr. of Connecticut, followed the precepts of Paracelsus. Winthrop practiced medicine himself and created drugs of his own design based on Paracelsian and alchemical principles.[4]

Despite these changes, most medical practitioners in both England and America still practiced under the ancient Galenic humoral paradigm. That is, they believed that illness was caused by an imbalance of one of the body's four humors: blood, black bile (melancholy), yellow bile (choler), and phlegm. Each humor was associated with a certain temperature and element: blood was hot and moist and associated with the element air, black bile was cold and dry and corresponded to the element of earth; yellow bile was hot and dry and corresponded with fire; and phlegm was cold and wet and associated with water. No person, even when healthy, had a perfect balance of the humors. In everyone, one or two humors dominated the others, creating temperamental differences. The language of humoral medicine is still with us in words that describe mood or temperament: *sanguine, melancholy, choleric, phlegmatic*. The predominant humor in each individual predisposed him or her to certain kinds of illnesses.[5]

Many things, from a sudden chill to an emotional shock to a poorly digested meal, could cause a humoral imbalance. Other diseases could arise from foul air or miasma, which could also upset the humoral balance or otherwise poison the system. This concept of disease was markedly different from the one we use today, in two ways. First, in the Galenic system, disease arose from the human body itself, rather than from outside forces. Second, there were no "specific" diseases, only unbalanced humors. One disease could transmute into another as the proportion of each humor changed. While the early modern English recognized and named different ailments such as plague and smallpox, they described particular sets of symptoms rather than disease entities. Some sophisticated physicians in England were beginning to move away from this paradigm, and to name and classify diseases based on clinical observation. However, these ideas were not universally accepted even by physicians, and among lay-folk they were virtually unknown.[6] Most early modern people "did not think in terms of an underlying invasive entity with specific, determinate, and persisting identity," as we do today.[7]

Medical therapies, whether prescribed by a learned member of the Royal College of Physicians or an illiterate colonial housewife, were aimed at restoring humoral balance. Galenic herbalists such as Nicholas Culpeper classified herbs by humoral qualities. One chapter of Culpeper's famous herbal begins, "Herbs, Plants and other medicines manifestly operate by Heat, Coldness, Dryness or Moisture; for the World being composed of so many Qualities, they and they only can be found in the world."[8] Culpeper then goes on to classify plants according to this system, giving the exact degree of temperature and dryness belonging to each plant. Galenic medicine worked by identifying the illness and prescribing herbal mixtures that would counterbalance the nature of the disease. That is, if a disease originated from a cold, moist humor, the practitioner would prescribe a mixture of hot, dry herbs. Most medicines were also designed to drive out superfluous humors. Thus, emetics, purges, diaphoretics, and other expulsive drugs were the most common kinds of medicines.[9]

While Galenic herbal remedies dominated practice, a growing number of elite physicians were beginning to follow the teachings of Paracelsus. Paracelsian theory differed from Galenic theory in two ways: Paracelsus believed in distinct diseases, as opposed to unbalanced humors, and he advocated the use of chemical drugs in addition to herbs. Paracelsus mixed his medical ideas with a dose of Christian mysticism, believing that the human body is presided over by a partly physical, partly spiritual soul that controls movement, sense, and thought. Paracelsus's ideas were particularly popular among Puritan physicians, who saw his theories as a Christian alternative to the "pagan" paradigm of ancient Greeks and Romans like Hippocrates and Galen. Paracelsian physicians such as John Winthrop Jr. introduced compounds based on lead, sulfur, and mercury to New England.[10]

Other aspects of Paracelsian medicine were beginning to creep into the dominant Galenic paradigm. For instance, practitioners began to use the so-called doctrine of similars when choosing drugs. This doctrine was as old as Hippocrates but was revived by Paracelsus. The doctrine can be summarized by the phrase "like is cured by like." That is, the cure for a disease could be recognized by the similarity of the appearance of the plant, animal, or mineral to the symptoms of the disease. Thus, the bright yellow herb saffron was a good cure for jaundice (which tints the skin and eyes yellow), and kidney beans were beneficial for urinary tract disorders. This theory was widely adopted by popular healers, even by those who had never heard of the rest of Paracelsus's ideas. Despite the differences in theory between the two systems, in practice Paracelsian medicine relied as heavily on purgatives and emetics as Galenic medicine did. Most practitioners were not doctrinaire. They continued to use Galenic herbal remedies and merely incorporated chemical and "signature" drugs into an eclectic practice.[11]

Just as the early modern concepts of disease and healing were very different from ours, when a colonial American said a medicine "worked kindly," he or she meant something different from what we would mean. An effective medicine was one that had visible results— that is, the expulsion of large amounts of humors. As a result, most people expected to feel much worse after taking physick. Emetics caused nausea and vomiting; purges and enemas could cause painful cramps.[12] Patients tolerated the discomfort in the hope of a cure—or at the very least, an improvement—in the long run. Both patients and practitioners kept track of the quantity and quality of excretions in minute detail: "[The medicine] wraught 1st by stoole, which was not loose, a good while after, he had a pretty large vomit: after that, a small stoole not very loose: after that another litle one very loose."[13] To the author of this passage, this was a description of a very effective drug.

Practitioners of all kinds shared these concepts of disease and healing. Popular and learned concepts of disease and healing "merged together into a largely amorphous whole."[14] With this shared body of knowledge, the relationship between patients and healers was much more egalitarian than it would later become, since most ordinary people had enough medical knowledge to make informed choices about their care and to judge critically the care they received.[15]

As a result, the medical system of seventeenth-century England was a "medical marketplace" with a large number of different kinds of practitioners available. The patient could choose from any of the following: licensed members of the Royal College of Physicians in London; apothecaries, who diagnosed as well as prescribed; barber-surgeons, including those who specialized in one kind of surgery, such as removing bladder stones or setting broken bones; so-called "empiric" physicians, who scorned a university education in favor of learning based on experience; midwives, both licensed and unlicensed; and men and women known as "cunning folk," whose practices included spells and charms as well as cordials and poultices. Patients chose their practitioner according to their financial means and personal inclinations.

In both England and the American colonies, this situation was intensified by the lack of learned physicians. In London there was only one learned practitioner for every four thousand people. Outside of the city, the situation was worse. Even potential patients who could devote time and money to consulting a learned doctor were restricted by poor travel conditions. Therefore, for the vast majority of English people, including the wealthy and titled, medical care came from a practitioner without a formal education or license. In the colonies, this situation replicated itself in a more extreme form.[16]

Given the widely disseminated lay knowledge of medicine, the variations in training of practitioners, and the lack of the most elite practitioners, it is not surprising that learned (usually male) and lay (often female) medical practices in New England were very similar, and that the two traditions overlapped. Consider, for example, these two recipes to cure hemorrhoids, the first from a manuscript book of recipes kept by women of the Brigham family of Massachusetts, the second from the commonplace book of the physician Thomas Palmer:

> Take a pounde of boares grease, 8 handfulls of Sage, a pounde of fresh butter, chope ye sage small, & set all on ye fire, wth 4 ounces of wax & let boyle . . . straine it through a coarse cloth into a gallipott, & when you use it, spread it upon browne paper so bigge as ye soareness, . . . yn lay on ye plaister & at ye first dress it twice a day.[17]

> Rx. Fresh butter, oyl of roses, of each 1 oz. . . . [and] white lead, washed., grind them in a mortar for an unguent. If ye

pain be vehement, take the yolk of an egg, oyle of roses, Juice of poppy or henbane.[18]

Both recipes use herbs, and both make ointments out of household ingredients like butter and eggs. Palmer's recipe calls for lead, showing a familiarity with Paracelsian medicine that the Brighams did not have. Other than that, the recipes are very similar.

GENDER, RANK, AND EARLY AMERICAN
REDICAL PRACTICE

Both men and women practiced medicine in colonial New England. Just as in England, the variety of practitioners created a medical marketplace of physicians, midwives, surgeons, and other healers. Patients were not doctrinaire in choosing who would care for them. The sick called different practitioners to perform different services— a midwife for childbirth, a male surgeon for removing a tumor.

A few practices traditionally were performed by only one sex. Women dominated midwifery and the care of pregnant women. Men were rarely, if ever, called to cases of childbirth in the seventeenth century, and while the male presence would increase over time, midwives continued to practice well into the nineteenth century. In addition to attending births, midwives also took care of various female reproductive problems.

Similarly, only men performed bleedings. The medical records of male practitioners contain many references to the practice. Dr. John Barton charged a shilling to bleed a man for an "aching humor" in 1679. Thomas Palmer included elaborate rules for bleeding in his commonplace book and recorded using the technique on two of his patients. (Palmer also noted that bleeding killed one of them!)[19] In contrast, the Brigham women's medical recipe book has no references at all to bleeding. Perhaps the most telling piece of evidence is the following entry from Ebenezer Parkman's diary:

[September] 28 [1757] Mrs. Tainter yesterday brot & applyd a Tobacco Ointment to my Wifes Legg—but it is no better.

29, Dr. Chace bleeds my wife.[20]

The Parkmans called in two practitioners in this case—a woman, Mrs. Tainter, to apply a poultice, and a man, Dr. Chase, to let blood. The Parkmans consulted a variety of healers over the years, including a number of women. However, on the twenty-eight occasions that Ebenezer wrote that a family member had been bled, a male practitioner performed the procedure every time.[21]

Why bloodletting was performed exclusively by men is not entirely clear. It seems likely that a combination of factors was involved. It may be significant that bleeding was thought to be dangerous for small children and pregnant women—groups that looked primarily to female practitioners. Perhaps midwives and nurses rarely performed the procedure because there was little call for it in their practices. Bloodletting was also closely associated with other kinds of men's work. Some phlebotomists were surgeons, and many surgeons learned their skill during military service. Training as a military surgeon would teach a man to distinguish between veins and arteries—an essential distinction in performing bleedings, if the patient were to survive the procedure. Men also did most of the slaughtering and butchering of large animals, a practice that would provide a certain amount of anatomical knowledge as well as an opportunity to practice quick and efficient techniques for opening veins.[22]

Despite the male domination of bleeding and surgery and the female domination of midwifery and female complaints, most medical services could be provided by a practitioner of either sex. At times, a sick person might consult two or three different healers during the course of an illness. Patients and healers perceived several categories of practitioners. Patients used these categories to make their choices, and healers used them to define themselves and their practices.

Categories of medical practitioners were strongly hierarchical. As in England, position in this hierarchy was determined in part by the person's social rank, in part by education and training, and in part by gender. Women practitioners, in general, were ranked below men, although there was enough overlap between male and female practice to make the rankings ambiguous. Among males, social rank and education intertwined to create a ladder of practitioner levels. Healers of different ranks and genders often cooperated with each other in caring for their patients, but healers as well as the patients were very aware of the differences between them. The following brief profiles illustrate several broad categories of practitioners. While there were many gradations between categories, and many healers that did not fit neatly into one category or another, the healers described below illustrate the most common and most easily defined types. These men and women are typical of their practitioner type, and their names and practices will reappear in the pages that follow.

At the top, as in England, were the most learned physicians, men with a university degree. These practitioners were rare and very well respected by their communities and their patients. In general, these high-ranking men were leaders in their communities as a result of family connections, wealth, and education. Typical of this type of practitioner was John Winthrop Jr. Winthrop was the son of Governor John Winthrop of Massachusetts. The younger Winthrop had a similar career. He had a university education (although not a degree in medicine) and a number of intellectual and scientific interests. Like his father, he spent many years as governor of a colony—in his case, Connecticut.

Winthrop never supported himself as a physician. In fact, it is not even clear that he charged for his services. However, Winthrop did have a widespread practice. He invented his own medicines, based on Paracelsian and Galenic principles, and prescribed these medicines to a large number of patients. In general, his patients did not come to him to be examined and diagnosed, but instead communicated with him by letter. Most of these patients had already consulted other healers before writing to Winthrop. Often, Winthrop was the doctor of last resort—the physician who could offer hope for seemingly hopeless cases. For instance, the Leete family consulted Winthrop several times with regard to their daughter Graciana, who was born with a number of severe problems, including what appears to have been cerebral palsy. The Leetes begged Winthrop for help with Graciana's "trembling legs," noting that the women healers they had already consulted were baffled. Winthrop presented himself as a gentleman doctor, with all that that implies: he did not support himself with his practice, and perhaps most important, he did not work directly with his patients. Real gentlemen had other means of support and certainly did not work with their hands.[23]

Perhaps most important to his status, Winthrop presented himself as an intellectual, and his patients viewed him as such. His family status, his European education, and his membership in English learned societies all contributed to this image. New England was characterized by a "zeal for learning," and learned men garnered a great amount of respect. Medicine, science, theology, and other intellectual pursuits were highly valued throughout the Anglo-American world.[24] Education and learning were some of the attributes that defined a high-ranking gentleman, and maintaining "higher culture" was one of the duties of societal leaders. Respect for learning and respect for rank were deeply intertwined with respect for medicine. Even in a society like New England's, where basic literacy was relatively widespread, extensive learning was strongly associated with high social rank and political leadership. Latin education, in particular, had "the indisputable cachet of gentility."[25] For Winthrop, respect for intellectual achievement guaranteed his position at the top of the medical hierarchy.

More common were practitioners just below the lofty level of Winthrop. These men called themselves "doctor" or "physician" but did not have a university degree or a doctorate of medicine. Instead, they acquired their skill from a preceptor or "master." Such an apprenticeship would have been much like other training for skilled work. The apprentice accompanied the master on his rounds, to observe and assist; he helped the master prepare medicines; and he did general work in the master's household. If the master owned a set of medical books, the apprentice would read them, and perhaps memorize long passages or copy portions into a personal notebook.[26] Despite not having been to a university, such doctors were literate and conversant with learning. John Barton of Essex County, Massachusetts, represents this group.

Barton's account book reveals much about his attitudes toward both medical practice and medical learning. The first ten pages or so are medical recipes and instructions. Both the recipes and the notes are a combination of learned and folk traditions. Barton dedicated several pages of his commonplace book to a lengthy description of the uses of urine in diagnosing illness. The language of the uroscopy segment suggests that Barton may have copied these instructions from a book, or taken them down as dictation from a preceptor: "In u[rine] many things are to be considered. 1. the quantity 2 the regions . . . , then the 20 colours and the 20 contents, and what al they doth signify." Such language is the mark of a learned practice. Yet a few pages earlier, he noted that a "rost Turnop" applied to a patient's body relieves pain. Practices like this one clearly come from a lay tradition of healing.[27]

Barton's practice was similarly balanced between gentlemanly intellectual practice and the hard daily work of an artisan. Barton taught local boys to read and write and wrote letters and other documents for illiterate patients. He also made an attempt at scientific observation, keeping track of cloud formations for a few days and commenting on the weather. At the same time, it was clear that his practice was much more direct than that of John Winthrop Jr. He supervised the dosing of his patients with "vomits" and pills and monitored the effects. He depended on patient fees to support himself and often accepted honey, wool, or meat in lieu of cash. In other cases, he was forced to dun patients for months or even take them to court in order to collect his bills. Barton was by no means a low-status man—he is referred to as "Mr." Barton in the Essex County records, for instance—but neither was he as high ranking as Winthrop.

A final class of practitioner filled the bottom of the hierarchy. This group consisted of healers who had little formal training and who practiced only sporadically. Daniel Ela, also of Essex County, falls into this category. He was most often identified as a tanner or leather worker, but like most men of the time he dabbled in other trades, including innkeeping and trading in lumber and other goods. Medical care seemed to have been another of his sidelines. A Newbury family called on Ela to dress the injured leg of a servant in 1674. In the same year, Richard Langhorne's probate inventory records that Langhorne owed Ela one pound and nine pence for unspecified medical care. Like many female healers, Ela served as an assistant to other, higher-ranking practitioners. In the case of the servant with the injured leg, Ela was following the instructions of a middle-level practitioner, John Dole. It seems probable that there were many informal practitioners like Ela, or others who specialized in one kind of care, like bloodletting or setting bones.[28]

Social rank was not the only determinant of one's position in the medical hierarchy. Gender also played its part and complicated the categories. One major difference between men and women is that there were not any female practitioners with the same "gentlemanly" kind of practice as John Winthrop Jr. All women practitioners worked directly with patients, dirtying their hands and clothing with medicines and bodily fluids, and none of them had the same ambitions toward scientific inquiry as high-level men did. The actual practice of women healers remained consistent from practitioner to practitioner, regardless of rank. The distinctions between women healers were primarily related to social status. Women of higher social rank tended to have more patients and to garner more respect than did their lower-ranking peers.

At the top were women of prominent families, whose access to education was better than that of most women, and whose social authority was unquestioned. Ann Hutchinson falls into this category. While Hutchinson's historical legacy stems mostly from her religious ideas and power struggle with John Winthrop Sr., her contemporaries knew her as a healer first, before they knew her as a theologian. Hutchinson "was one of those high-status women whose expertise in health care in general and childbirth in particular was greatly valued in the early settlements."[29] Her social status was unquestioned. She was the daughter of a minister and the wife of a wealthy merchant. While we know little of her actual education, it is clear from the course of her life and her performance at her trials that at the very least, she was a well-read woman. In addition, she made her fame (or notoriety) through her theological innovations and religious leadership—areas usually associated with those who had a higher education. All of these factors came together to make her as close to a female intellectual as Massachusetts had. As with intellectuals like John Winthrop Jr., Hutchinson's educational level added an air of authority to her prescriptions.

Other, less prominent women were well-regarded healers. Anna Gott Brigham Maynard of Marlborough, Massachusetts, was a respected healer among her immediate neighbors. Maynard's first husband's family was one of the leading families of her rural area. Both the Brighams and the Maynards were large landholders, and the men of both families held a variety of local offices. Her first husband, Samuel Brigham, was a physician, of the same "middling" rank as John Barton. Her second was known his whole life as "Captain Maynard" because of his militia rank. Maynard herself clearly had considerable skills, and it is possible that she may have learned some of them from her first husband or from the women of his family. The local minister, Ebenezer Parkman, sought her advice for his rheumatism (she prescribed garlic steeped in rum). She was also the practitioner called in to care for a "poor sick woman" who had fallen ill while traveling to join her husband.[30] While not as well educated or as high ranking as Ann Hutchinson, Maynard did have enough status in the local community to be called in for difficult cases and to give advice to families other than her own.

At the bottom of the hierarchy for women practitioners was the vast array of ordinary housewives, each with her own skills and her own collection of pet remedies. These women generally tended to their own families and to their neighbors but did not have the special abilities, education, or social status that raised some women healers above others.

The medical practices of men and women often overlapped, and patients often consulted both. When Ebenezer Parkman fell ill with "greiv'd Nausea and freqt reaching vomits," he sent first for Dr. Chase, a male practitioner. Chase declared that Parkman had "the jaundice." Upon receiving this diagnosis, Parkman immediately sent his son to a female practitioner, Mrs. Kimball, for a dose of her "Remedy." Parkman felt much better the next day and ate "with relish" for the first time in several days. Chase and Kimball played different but equally important parts in Parkman's treatment.[31]

Similarly, many women incorporated into their own recipe notebooks the medical recipes given to them by men, such as "A receipt for ye stone used by Mr. Paule Parke minister of Peterborrough," which should be taken "wn yu finde any grudging of ye stone . . . 4 or 5 spoonefulls of it in white wine." Housewives also recorded recipes from doctors, such as "Doctor Craggs direction for fitts of ye winde & off the mother." Male practitioners, even physicians, were not so lofty that women wouldn't dare to use their remedies; nor did physicians hold themselves aloof from female practitioners.[32]

Given these broad areas of overlap in practice, it is sometimes difficult to see what difference gender made in medical matters. However, it is clear that practitioners and patients believed there were important differences. Healers defined themselves and their practices in a gendered way. In general, male practitioners presented themselves as intellectual practitioners, and their skills were seen as cerebral ones. Women healers, on the other hand, were most often perceived as having practical, empirical skills. Patients who consulted more than one practitioner often chose men when mental skill was required and women for day-to-day care and medicines. In consulting Dr. Chase and Mrs. Kimball, Ebenezer Parkman made such a choice. Chase made the diagnosis, based on his education; Kimball made the medicine to cure the jaundice Chase had identified. Such subtle gender differences not only influenced the way patients chose practitioners, but also were very much a part of the way healers thought of themselves. One way these different self-images manifested themselves is in the ways male and female practitioners kept records of their practices.

John Winthrop Jr.'s medical journal is very different from women's notebooks. Winthrop's journal contains medical records, rather than a set of recipes. Each of the entries describes the illness of a particular patient and records the medicines he concocted as a cure. Some of Winthrop's notes are in plain English; the remainder, including the ingredients of each medicine, are recorded in a combination of alchemical and astronomical symbols, used in a way that had meaning to him but are difficult for an outsider to interpret. Winthrop was so good at keeping his recipes to himself that the ingredients of his pet remedy, rubila, remain uncertain.

John Winthrop was not unique in keeping his medical records in code. Thomas Palmer of Plymouth, a middle-level physician, also recorded many of his personal medical recipes and other information in an idiosyncratic shorthand that used phonetic symbols for words and syllables. Palmer's shorthand was based on a 1690 system that he changed significantly to suit his own purposes. The notebook remained unreadable until Thomas Rogers Forbes broke the code.[33]

Winthrop's and Palmer's journals were meant to be private—even secret. Palmer went so far as to title his journal "The Admirable Secrets of Physick and Chyrurgery [surgery]." But the word *secrets* had several meanings in the seventeenth century. In the Elizabethan world, one meaning was "specific and infallible remedies."[34] It seems very likely that this was one of the resonances of the word for both Palmer and Winthrop. Winthrop's personal remedies were in great demand. His medicine rubila, in particular, was requested for a variety of ailments.

Connected to this notion of secrets as infallible remedies was the idea that each physician must have his own theory of disease. Men with scientific ambitions, like Palmer and Winthrop, based their self-definition as scientists on creating their own "grand theory," which would produce its own infallible remedies. As Palmer wrote on the title page of his notebook, "Foelix qui potuit rerum cognoscere Causas," meaning "Fortunate is he who can understand the causes of things."[35] The seventeenth century was a time when several theories of disease were competing for ascendancy. Each theory had its proponents and detractors, and passions on this subject often ran high. Physicians were classified according to the theory they followed: was he an iatrochemist or an iatromechanist? Or was he a traditional Galenist? That is, did he believe that bodily processes were analogous to chemical reactions or to the workings of machines? Or did he cling to the ancient humoral theory of sickness?

Winthrop is not explicit about his theory in his medical notebooks, but it is well known that he was greatly interested in iatrochemistry. His personal library contained literature on the subject, and he corresponded for years with European adherents of iatrochemical theory. His use of chemical drugs and his predilection for chemical symbols in his journal suggest that his practice was deeply influenced by the theory.[36]

The word *secret* also has meaning in the context of Palmer's and Winthrop's remedies. Palmer and Winthrop kept their journals in a system of writing that very few, if any, would understand. The code functioned as both shorthand and as a device for keeping the "secrets" truly secret. The idea that medical and scientific knowledge should be private knowledge had ancient origins. Through the medieval period, tradition had it that God revealed the workings of nature to a select few. The knowledge belonged to them alone, and if it was revealed to the "vulgar," the knowledge would be corrupted and rendered invalid, even dangerous. While this kind of scientific secrecy was fading in the early modern period, it was a likely influence in Winthrop's and Palmer's decisions to keep their notebooks in code.[37]

In the late sixteenth and early seventeenth centuries, a new "secrets" tradition established itself. Knowledge was no longer the property of the individual sage. Instead it belonged to scientific communities. These groups shared knowledge among themselves and used the possession of knowledge to define themselves as gentlemen and scholars. Winthrop, in particular, seems to have designed his record-keeping system with this purpose in mind. Although his code had the effect of rendering his records unreadable to many, the kind of code he chose reflects the assumed audience for his work. Winthrop used alchemical and astronomical symbols, symbols that a learned contemporary would have recognized immediately. Even if the reader could not interpret the entire meaning of the passage, the symbols defined Winthrop's audience as that of the community of scientists.

After the Baconian revolution in scientific thinking, with its emphasis on making knowledge public, scientific communities still maintained a tight grip over the distribution of knowledge. The Royal Society in London, dedicated to the "publication" of scientific knowledge, still clung to the ethos that such knowledge had to be kept among those who knew how to use it. Even "public" knowledge had to be presented to a strictly defined "public"—carefully screened, appropriately educated gentlemen. Such a restriction meant that members of the society were the ones who defined scientific knowledge. In doing so, scientific societies maintained another function of scientific secrecy: the consolidation of power and social status. Starting in the seventeenth century, "the secrets of nature are more the monopoly of an autonomous corporation of specialists than ever before. The cultural function of secrecy is to articulate a boundary, to circumscribe an interior that is off limits to outsiders, to mark off a sphere of autonomous power."[38] In this context, it is significant that women were excluded from membership in these learned societies. While women healers were commonplace in both England and the colonies, their absence from the scientific public reserved the highest medical rank for men.

Thus, Winthrop's and Palmer's notebooks contained secrets in several senses of the word. They contained infallible remedies, based on their own theories of causes, and they contained scientific knowledge that could be revealed only to certain carefully defined audiences. Both of these kinds of secrets were crucial to the men's self-definition as insiders, gentlemen, and scientists. Such a definition was particularly important to John Winthrop Jr., who was the only colonial to be elected to the Royal Society in London.

Women's medical documents are very different. Women in the Brigham family in Massachusetts kept a medical notebook of their own. It contains transcriptions of hundreds of medicinal recipes, passed down through four generations. This was not a "secret" document—quite the opposite. The keepers of the notebook always gave proper credit to the person who gave them the recipe. The way the recipes are transcribed reflects a system of shared knowledge. In this respect, the Brigham notebook reflects the way in which women practiced medicine. A woman, even an educated, intellectual woman like Ann Hutchinson, saw medicine as a skill to be shared. Many men, even middling men like Thomas Palmer, saw medicine as an intellectual discipline, accessible only to the educated few.

Page from the Brigham family medical notebook. This notebook is a unique document illustrating the way women shared medical knowledge among themselves. Note that the authors indicate the source of each recipe. (Courtesy, American Antiquarian Society.)

Nor are there references in the Brigham notebook to a "grand theory" of disease. Medical theory is implied throughout, woven in between the instructions and recipes, but nowhere is there a section on the root cause of all diseases or the basis for all cures. While the men's documents have, to a greater or lesser extent, a theoretical orientation, the Brigham notebook has a decidedly empirical bent. Women's medical practice was a household skill. Thus, the Brigham notebook emphasizes the practical rather than the theoretical. Tried and true family recipes were the core of their knowledge, rather than abstract ideas about the cause of disease and the workings of nature.

This empirical orientation puts the Brigham notebook into another tradition of "secrets" literature. Some European practitioners rebelled against the elitism and arcane traditions of academic medicine and science and made a point of revealing the "secrets of nature." These practitioners often sold their medicines and recipes to the public at large at fairs and town markets. Lying behind their practices was an assumption that the workings of nature were ultimately incomprehensible, but that human beings could use nature's secrets to their own advantage. Their published recipes took advantage of these "hidden" causes to create dye, ink, metal tools, and medicines. While most of the recipes in the Brigham notebook came from female relatives, a number were copied from *Digby's Closet*, a recipe book in this "secrets" tradition. This concept of the secrets of nature had a greater resonance with women's day-to-day practice than did theoretical concerns. When a housewife gave willow bark to a child and lowered a fever, it was more like harnessing an incomprehensible force than seeking forbidden knowledge.[39]

There is another, more subtle distinction between the records kept by men and those kept by women. These records reflect not just differences in medical practice, but differences of gender and rank identity. The Brigham women were unusual in that they wrote their recipes down. Very few women were able to write at all, although most could read. At the time, the ability to write had social meaning. Race and religion were closely linked to literacy. Native Americans were taught to read and write only as part of religious conversion; enslaved Africans were not taught to read at all. The possession of such skills was not universal but the trait of a specific group: white Christians. The ability to write and create such documents helped distinguish a specific, dominant community, a "community of learning whereby ... status as civilized Christians was defined."[40] Those excluded from literacy, for whatever reason, were aware that they were also excluded from the power that accrued to the literate.[41]

Reading and writing defined not just race and status but gender as well. Writing was associated with male occupations, most specifically the ministry and commerce. Like Native Americans and Africans, women were defined in part by their lack of access to writing and print. Just as books and letters defined a white community, the creation of books, letters, and written records defined a community that was predominantly male.[42]

Even within the community of those who could write, there were social distinctions. The specific kind of handwriting a person used was another important social marker. Merchants used one kind of handwriting; ministers, another; women, another. A person reading a document would know how to interpret not just the text but the social status of the writer: "The appropriate degree of authority granted to the handwritten word . . . was inscribed into the very words themselves."[43] Such a meaning is evident in the different hands used by Winthrop and "A.W.," the main compiler of the Brigham notebook who identified herself only by initials. Winthrop used the so-called court hand. The court hand was an older style, going out of fashion in the seventeenth century. True to its name, it remained associated with legal documents and other court business. Usually, only boys were taught to use this style of handwriting. The court hand implied an old-fashioned education, male gender, and a high social status. A.W. used the "secretary hand." This style was used by both men and women, but unlike the court hand, it was a "workmanlike" handwriting, associated with merchants and other middling classes. It did not carry the social cachet of the court hand, or the "italic hands" that were just coming into fashion. Thus, a mere glance at the Brigham and Winthrop documents would have told a seventeenth-century observer much about the authors.[44]

If handwriting was a marker of both social identity and power, male physicians used their handwritten journals to mark themselves as powerful. Just as alchemical symols helped exclude the "vulgar," the use of code and shorthand functioned as a kind of "superliteracy," a handwriting style even less accessible than ordinary script. Women and lesser men could not read these men's secrets. Instead, the documents marked membership in an exclusive club, a club made up of educated, high-status men like themselves. Just as the language of the Bible defined a community of "white Christians" against other communities of enslaved Africans and pagan Indians, so did Winthrop's and Palmer's shorthand define a community of elite male physicians against other communities of lesser male practitioners and women.

The Brigham women were excluded from this elite group, but their document defines their practice against both male and female healers who were illiterate. The Brigham family, which included several important female practitioners such as Anna Brigham Maynard and Hepzibah Brigham Maynard, was thus a level above most other women practitioners in the layers of rank, even if the Brighams were below male physicians in the layers of gender. By writing their recipes down, the Brigham women also defined themselves as part of a restricted community. The vast majority of practitioners, both male and female, left no written records of their own. They had no secrets to defend and no literacy to help them lay claim to remedies and theories. Both the Brigham women and men like Palmer and Winthrop rated themselves against this group, and used writing and literacy to define themselves in relation to them. Medical practice and medical knowledge were thus inextricably linked to definitions of community, social hierarchy, and gender. All three of these institutions were crucial concerns of seventeenth-century New Englanders. These themes, and the ways they intersected at the bedsides of the sick, will be central to the chapters that follow.

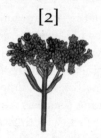

Called to the Bedside

Medicine in the Household

ON A RAINY LATE SEPTEMBER day, Anna Cromwell added another log to her fire. Next to the hearth was a pallet bed, made up with the heaviest coverlets. Cromwell's oldest daughter was in bed recovering from a flux with fever. She was well enough to sit up but very weak. What she needs, Cromwell thought, is a bowl of sack posset.

Cromwell knew the recipe by heart, but she still consulted the family recipe book before she got out her spices and wine. Her sister's cordial for the flux had saved her daughter's life. Now, Cromwell turned to her cousin's recipe for posset: "Take 10 eggs, whites and yolks," it began. Cromwell had only four eggs. They would have to do. She beat them with a dribble of sack wine and a pinch of nutmeg, warming the mixture slowly over a basin of coals. The key, she had learned, is to add the milk in a very thin stream as you beat the eggs—an important point she has written in the margin of the recipe book. After Cromwell's daughter drank the posset, Cromwell thought she looked a little better.[1]

Women like Anna Cromwell practiced medicine every day. Ordinary housewives performed a range of tasks that we might call medical practice: diagnosing illnesses, prescribing and making medicines, and providing support and comfort to the sick. Such work was the domain of the mistress of the household. Even when a family called upon a more formally trained practitioner, the woman of the house made up his prescriptions and carried out his instructions. In early New England, medicine was an integral part of women's household work.

The accessibility of medical knowledge and the lack of elite male physicians created ideal conditions for widespread female medical practice in the New England colonies. When a person fell ill, the first and only practitioner likely to be called was the mistress of the household, armed with her knowledge of humors and herbs. Indeed, many medical tasks grew out of other kinds of women's work. The growing, preservation, and preparation of medicinal herbs was much the same as the growing, preservation, and preparation of foodstuffs. Nursing and watching at bedsides grew out of child care, and like the care of small children, was often delegated to adolescent daughters. Women treated medical knowledge not as a mysterious and difficult science but as an everyday art. Armed with these medical traditions, a housewife could feel confident about treating many kinds of illnesses.

Most women probably acquired their expertise through word of mouth, and the process is therefore lost to historians. Luckily, the Brigham family recipe book represents an astonishingly complete record of one family's medical knowledge and how it was spread from woman to woman, and from generation to generation.

The Brigham family recipe book probably originated in England in the early seventeenth century. The first page is inscribed "Anna Cromwell, my book of Receipts, December the 23th 1650"; however, Cromwell was not the first author. The transcriber of most of the recipes in the book was a woman who signed herself only with her initials: A.W; A.W. and Anna Cromwell were sisters. The book probably entered the Brigham family through Elizabeth Howe Brigham, who lived in Marlborough, Massachusetts, in the late seventeenth century. The next names inscribed in the book are those of Elizabeth's son, Charles Brigham, and his wife, Mary Peters Brigham. The book finally ended up in the hands of their daughter, Mary Brigham Parks, and her sister-in-law, Sarah Sartell Prentice.[2] All of these women contributed to the book. The Brigham recipe book thus represents the collective wisdom of four generations of women. It also demonstrates how women passed their knowledge on—from sister to sister, from mother-in-law to daughter-in-law, from sister-in-law to sister-in-law.

The authors of the recipe book kept a meticulous record of the origin of their recipes. There is an attribution for each recipe—whether for medicine, dye, wine, or food. The mysterious A.W. was particularly meticulous about recording the origins of her recipes. Most were from female kin, but unrelated women and men also contributed. One folder of the manuscript contains medical recipes A.W. attributed to thirty-four different women. The list includes relatives—sisters, aunts, cousins, daughters, and nieces—as well as a number of unrelated people. The nonrelatives represent a wide section of social rank. Some are referred to by their names without a courtesy title ("Bess Holmes"); others, with titles ranging from "Mistress" and "Madam" to "My Lady." Sometimes A.W. gave a "genealogy" for a recipe: "this receipt was given to my mother; from whom my aunt price had it whoe gave it to mee. A.W."[3] A.W. was clearly a particularly enthusiastic recipe collector, but the long list of names in the manuscript indicates that most women had a rich knowledge of healing. A young girl learned medicine not only from her mother but also from her female kin and neighbors.

Women also took advantage of learned medicine. A.W.'s recipes include a fair number that she attributed to physicians. Yet there was not a clear distinction between the medicines made by the likes of Anna Cromwell and Lucy English and those made by Dr. King. As we have seen, elite physicians and ordinary housewives shared a medical paradigm and used similar cures.

The making of medicines was virtually indistinguishable from cooking and food preparation. Seventeenth-century printed cookbooks published recipes for food and medicines together, sometimes in separate chapters, sometimes not. One 1653 cookbook printed recipes for "a maid dish of hartechoakes" and "an excellent medicine or salve for an ache" on the same page.[4] The Brigham notebook contains hundreds of handwritten recipes, from "A Frickasee of chickins" to "Directions for prevention in the time of the Plague." Sometimes the recipes themselves make no distinction between food and medicine. One example begins, "To preserve greene medlers wch are exellent good & case of looseness [of the bowels]." At the end of the recipe, the author wrote, "You may eate them as a sweetemeate also."[5] In the humoral paradigm, food and medicines were sometimes indistinguishable: the proper "heating" or "cooling" diet was as important to an invalid's prognosis as the proper purging drug.[6] The good housewife kept her family in health through her cooking as well as her cordials and salves.

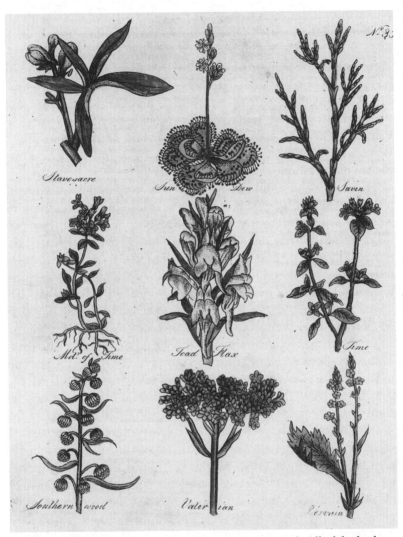

Plate from Nicholas Culpeper, *Herbal* (1634; 1813 reprint). All of the herbs illustrated here had medicinal uses. The plant in the upper-right corner is savin, which was commonly used to treat "obstructed menses" and to induce abortion. (Yale University, Harvey Cushing/John Hay Whitney Medical Library.)

For most illnesses, a housewife made herbal medicines with ingredients she had grown herself. Prescriptive literature made knowledge of herbs an essential trait of the efficient household mistress. "She must know all herbs," wrote Gervase Markham, in his household advice book, *The English Housewife*. "She shall also know the time of yeere, Moneth, and Moone in which all herbs are to be sowne; and when they are at their best flourishing, that gathering all Hearbs in their height of goodnesse, shee may have the prime use of the same."[7] When a woman planted a kitchen garden, it was sure to include medicinal plants among the carrots and peas.

The travel writer John Josselyn saw medicinal plants such as sorrel, marigolds, anise, and houseleeks growing in seventeenth-century New England gardens. Other plants Josselyn mentioned were primarily culinary herbs but had secondary uses as medicines: sage, coriander, thyme, and parsley.[8] Plants such as these—and many others Josselyn did not describe—turn up frequently in medicinal recipes. Elizabeth Davenport made a clyster, or enema, for her son that contained "anis seeds, fennell seedes, and a good handfull of Mallowes."[9] All of these ingredients could easily have come from her garden.

To be sure the herbs were available when needed to make into medicines, a housewife had to gather and preserve them properly. She had to harvest the plants at the right time of year, when they were at the peak of potency. "It is meete that our housewife know that from the eight of the Kalends of the moneth of Aprill, unto the eight of the Kalends of Iuly, all manner of hearbes and leaves are in that time most in strength and of the greatest virtue to be used and put in all manner of medicines," wrote Gervase Markham.[10] Herbs also had to be picked when the moon was in the right phase and the planets were in the right position. Almanacs often printed lists of propitious days for gathering plants. Leeds's almanac for 1693 declared June 13, 14, and 27 as the best days for harvesting roses, cinquefoil, carnations, and sage, since on those days Jupiter would have a positive influence on their potency.[11]

The simplest way to preserve medicinal plants was to dry them, preferably in the shade to retain their volatile oils. For some kinds of plants, however, this treatment was not appropriate. For instance, one recipe taken from the Brigham notebook recommends pickling as the best method for preserving elderflowers. Elderflowers were a mild laxative and induced sweating in persons with fever. They also had a diuretic effect, making them useful against kidney and bladder stones.[12] The flowers were best picked when the buds were just open. Once the flowers were picked and all extraneous materials such as stems, bark, and dirt were removed, the buds were boiled in a pan of "seething hot" water until "they be pritty well scalded." Next, the buds were drained in a "ryng sive," and salted. The amount of salt was up to the maker's discretion, though it was important that "you must not make them to[o] salte, they must have noe more salt in them but just to season them." When the flowers had cooled, they were put into a stone jar and covered with vinegar—"either sharpe beere vinegar or wine vinegar." Thus preserved, the elderflowers would keep indefinitely and be ready for use at any time.[13]

Sometimes herbs were made into medicines as soon as they were gathered. For this purpose, the best method was to extract the essence from the plants by "stilling" them: boiling the herbs in water or another liquid, then condensing the steam. Women made simple "waters" in this way, such as mint water and wormwood water. These herbal extracts were remedies for common ailments such as bellyache. Judging from the medicinal recipes in both printed and manuscript recipe books, stilling was by far the favored method for making herbs into medicines.[14]

Some of the recipes for stilled medicines were quite elaborate. One recipe contained twenty-seven ingredients and required three separate distillings at six-week intervals.[15] Most were simpler. This one is recommended for consumption: "Take 3 quarts of white wine & 3 [and a] halfe pounds of rosemary topps & still ye wine & rosemary together, let ye water droppe into a glasse wth suger in it, then take . . . a handfull of each, violets, rosemary, [and] wallflowers, putt them into ye distilled water & still them againe."[16] The dosage was one or two spoonfuls, every evening. An alternative method to stilling was infusion. A housewife could infuse herbs in water, wine, or beer by setting the mixture in the sun for a period of time. Both stilled and infused medicines could be sealed in small glazed earthenware pots (called "gallipots") and used when the need arose.

Not all medicines were made in advance. Enemas, poultices, salves, teas, and other concoctions were made on the spot. Many of the Brigham women's prescriptions for bruises and strains, for instance, called for fresh herbs. The plants were mixed into butter or suet that had been melted together with beeswax to make a salve. Similar substances were used for rashes, "the itch," and boils. In all likelihood, a housewife made up medicines for common illnesses in advance and preserved the rest of her herbs as dried plants or simple distilled waters to use when the need arose.

Knowing how to mix a clyster or still a cordial was only part of a housewife's medical expertise. A woman also needed to know when to use her medicines. Early American housewives diagnosed illnesses in addition to treating them. Most diagnoses came from careful observation of the patient's symptoms. Elizabeth Davenport of New Haven gave the following detailed description of her maidservant's ailment in 1654:

> She had paine in her leggs, with swelling, and paine in her back and head, with illnes in her stomack and grypings and stoppages, about a weeke before you came hither: then Dr. Choyse gave her a purge, after which she was better, but getting cold upon it, she was much as before, though somewhat lightsommer, yet her leggs swelled againe and so continue, more or less, ever since, they now pitt and will stand so, she hath not noted how long. She is troubled with wind and water in her stomake, yet she sleepes well and hath competent appetite and digestion.[17]

Not only is this a thorough description of the trouble, but also it makes subtle diagnostic judgments. Davenport noticed that the servant "took cold" from the purge, despite the temporary relief it provided. She also perceived that the maid's stomach pain stemmed specifically from "wind and water." Such sophistication was not unusual; indeed, Davenport's contemporaries took it for granted. In Essex County, Massachusetts, in 1686, a group of women came to court to testify about the health of their neighbor, Sarah Boynton. Ebenezer Browne had struck Sarah with a ladder. Sarah, who was pregnant, suffered great pain and sent for her neighbors. When they arrived, they found her in a terrible state: "Wee found the said Sarah Boynton wife of Joseph Bointon very full of paine like to Travel paines, & soe wee left her expecting that she would miscarry & did expect it dayly."[18] In making its decision regarding the fate of Browne, the court relied almost exclusively on the women's determination that Sarah would lose her baby.

Close observation of symptoms was the technique most women used to determine the cause and potential cure of an illness. Some women, however, had more sophisticated techniques at their disposal. Elizabeth Davenport, whose observation skills we have already seen, also practiced the venerable technique of uroscopy. A uroscopist observed the color, sediments, and other qualities of a patient's urine in order to diagnose an illness. The practice had been so widespread in medieval Europe that the urine flask was an instantly recognizable symbol of the physician, much as the stethoscope is today. By the seventeenth century, the practice had fallen into disfavor among the most elite physicians but was still common among other practitioners. It was so common, in fact, that in the early eighteenth century Cotton Mather still used the disparaging term "piss prophet" to refer to a physician.[19]

There are three references to Elizabeth Davenport's practice of uroscopy in her husband's letters. Once, she observed that her husband's urine was "high colored" with a "black settlement," which she thought might have been blood. The other two occasions took place during her son's serious illness in December of 1660. At the onset of the disease, John Jr.'s urine was "thickish and yellowish"; as he worsened, it turned "the colour of paler coloured oranges."[20] Unfortunately, John Davenport did not record how his wife interpreted her findings. It seems unlikely, though, that she would have made these observations without some idea of how to decipher them. Her diagnostic scheme was probably similar to that used by contemporary male physicians.[21]

Most care of the sick involved neither distilling medicines nor observing urine, however. The most time-consuming part of colonial medical care was "watching." Watching was just that—sitting at the bedside, getting the invalid a cup of beer, being on hand if he or she took a turn for the worse, saying a prayer with the sick person if he or she requested it. Watchers divided into shifts to ensure that someone was awake at the bedside all day and all night. Neighbors and kin came to assist the family in this task.

In general, anyone could do this work. While families who could afford it sometimes employed professional nurses, on the whole "watching" was a nonspecialized task. Men as well as women watched, but the job fell mostly to women. Both men and women sat with male patients; women almost exclusively sat with female patients. In many cases the long hours of bedside watching fell to adolescent girls.[22]

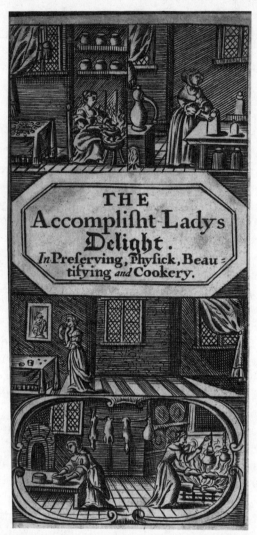

Title page from *The Accomplisht-Ladys Delight* (1683). This popular household manual, published in England, contains recipes for food and cosmetics as well as medicines. The woman in the upper-right corner is making a medicine; the object behind her is a still, set over the fire to boil. The woman to the left of her is grinding herbs or other materials with a mortar and pestle. The pictures below illustrate other feminine skills: beautifying oneself and cooking. These images illustrate that medical practice was an inherent part of a housewife's duties. (Beinecke Rare Book and Manuscript Library, Yale University.)

When small children were sick, however, their mothers did most of the watching, even during the all-night shifts usually handled by teenage girls. Mothers held their sick infants and toddlers on their laps or in their arms. Sometimes circumstances or their own health prevented mothers from caring for their children, but they preferred to do most of the watching themselves whenever they could. Elizabeth Mather sat up with a "languishing" child despite her own advanced pregnancy, and when she fell suddenly into labor, she delivered her baby at her son's bedside. Even when older children were sick or injured, their mothers sat up with them at night. When nine-year-old Billy Parkman cut himself badly while chopping wood, Hannah Parkman watched with him in case the bleeding started afresh.[23]

The household mistress had a deep obligation to care for all who lived under her roof, including servants. This obligation manifested itself in a disturbing way in a Newbury, Massachusetts, court case in 1674. Young Hugh March had been apprenticed to the Lowell family. Shortly after he moved into the Lowell household, he became quite sick. He developed a rash on his legs so severe that he had trouble walking, and became so weak that he could do nothing but lie on his pallet and cry. The Lowells wanted the Marches to take their son back until he recovered, but the Marches objected, insisting that the Lowells provide care. The most telling testimony in the case came from Judith March, Hugh's mother. In her deposition, she recounted a quarrel between herself and Goodwife Lowell. Judith March had gone to see her son at the Lowells' house. When she arrived, "his dame urged me to take him home, I was not willing & gave her reason for it." March said that the demands of the family tavern would prevent her from taking adequate care of her son. Goodwife Lowell replied, "Shee could not Attend him to goe upp & downe ye Staires."[24] Wherever Hugh spent his convalescence, the household mistress would bear primary responsibility for his care, and both women knew it. This dispute between two families concerning the care of a sick child originated as a dispute between women—those who would shoulder most of the burden if Hugh were placed in their household. While it is hard to sympathize with a mother who turned her back on a child who lay sobbing with pain on a corn husk mattress, the larger point is clear: medicine in the family was women's work.

It was easy, therefore, for some women to take their skills beyond the household. Perhaps the most well-known form of women's medical practice was midwifery. Midwives delivered babies, gave advice to pregnant women and new mothers, and were often consulted about the illnesses of newborn infants. In addition, midwives concerned themselves with all disorders of the female reproductive system. The midwife Goodwife Cooper tended Mrs. Thomas Pynchon when she had irregular and overly heavy periods. Similarly, when Molly Parkman developed an abscess in her breast while she was nursing, Mrs. Whitcomb lanced it.[25]

Some of midwives' skills stemmed from their special experience, but much of it grew naturally from household practice. Most housewives had a store of remedies for such maladies. The Brighams recorded recipes for irregular menses, "the whites" (possibly referring to a vaginal yeast infection), and postpartum "afterpains." This one, for threatened miscarriage, was passed on to one woman by her mother: "Take broth made of calves feet or knuckles of veale or any knitting thing; put in it shepards purse, knottgrasse, doves foote & rootes of red camphery, drink this 3 or 4 dayes & keep your selfe quiet."[26]

Other women took advantage of their household skills to establish themselves as paid healers. As we will see, these women were particularly skilled at nursing, bonesetting, and other forms of healing. Yet their skills differed from those of ordinary housewives more in degree than kind. The services that paid nurses and doctoresses offered were similar to those unpaid healers offered: special medicines, one-on-one "watching," and prescription diets. Women who did this kind of work usually took on chronic or difficult cases, perhaps because these patients had exhausted the medical resources of their families and were looking for help elsewhere. Patients could expect more attention, and perhaps a few skills that their female relations could not provide, such as minor surgery and bonesetting. Overall, however, the care of a doctoress would be familiar, and no doubt all the more comforting for that.

SCENARIOS OF HEALING: WOMEN AT THE BEDSIDE

How did all of these skills—diagnosis, medicine making, and watching—come together? It is possible to reconstruct the experience of both suffering and healing in early America, using women's documents and prescriptive literature. We have a pretty good idea how the women of the household would have responded when a person fell ill with a fairly serious illness, such as smallpox, measles, or even plague.[27]

First, they may well have tried to prevent it, especially if they knew a noxious disease was rampant in the neighborhood. Preventive measures involved strong-smelling substances to drive off the bad air: eating garlic, brimstone, or vinegar; smoking tobacco; or anointing the body with wormwood. If these measures failed, however, there were additional steps to take. When the first symptoms of a serious illness appeared, all authorities agreed that the best first step was to give the patient an emetic. Then, with a few exceptions, "as soon as yu have emptied ye stomake well . . . goe to bed and fitt yourselfe for sweate Lying in blanketts naked."[28] The housewife or main caretaker would build up the fire to a roar and prepare a diaphoretic medicine for the patient. Consistent with the humoral medicine paradigm, which involved driving humors out of the body, another first step was to cause sweating. A few diseases, most notably smallpox, did not lend themselves to this treatment. Smallpox was such a "hot" disease that excessive heat and sweating were thought dangerous. In general, however, sweating was part of the process of driving the disease from the body.

When the disease had established itself and seemed to be serious, the neighbors would begin to assemble. The patient would need watchers, and the household mistress would need help. This is when a skilled uroscopist used her skills, for the rest of the treatment depended on the nature of the disease—did it stem from a hot, cold, dry, or moist humor? Perhaps disputes broke out now, as different women might offer their pet remedies or rival uroscopists might argue over interpretations.

Meanwhile, teenage girls would set to work, making posset drink, or poached eggs, or jellied broth—the so-called easy foods thought best for the sick. These same girls would sit all night by the bedside, keeping the fire built up and piling more blankets on the patient to keep up the sweating. All the watchers would pray with the invalid and each other. If the illness started to turn for the worse, perhaps the local minister would pay a visit, to prepare the patient to meet God.

The primary tasks, however, revolved around the making of medicines appropriate to the disease. If the sickness involved a rash or other skin eruption, such as with smallpox or measles, it was important to "bring out" the sores. Suppressing them, it was believed, would drive the putrid humors inward and possibly kill the patient. In measles, for instance, humorally "hot" medicines were important to bring out the "hot" rash and purge the humors. Thus, hot-tasting herbs like ginger, steeped in scalding water and served as hot as the patient could bear, were appropriate treatment. In cases of suspected smallpox, if the pustules did not appear as expected, some practitioners applied blistering poultices, such as cantharides, to imitate and encourage a rash. If the sickness did not require such a purge through the skin, it almost certainly required some sort of purge: a clyster, emetic, or salivation.

Soon the disease would reach the crisis, the point when the patient showed signs of recovery or approaching death. The crisis, in Cotton Mather's words, "will often be attended with frightful circumstances; Grievous Oppression, Fainting, Vomiting, Purging and the Vapours, which is to say in one word, All that is terrible."[29] The watchers would wipe the patient's forehead, empty the chamber pots, change the linens if clean ones were to be had. If God willed it, the fever would break, and the sick person would be on the way back to health.

The convalescent period was much like the beginning of the illness. The watchers would cook and serve easy foods—gruel, broth, posset. Perhaps a few of the neighbors would begin to leave, and the nighttime shifts would be curtailed a bit. Some authors recommended one last series of purges after the worst of the sickness was over, to drive the last of the putrid humors away. The invalid would begin to get up and perhaps do simple tasks in the house. Finally, the last of the neighbors would go home, and everyone would return to their neglected chores and everyday life.

Childbirth followed a similar course.[30] When the very first signs of labor began to appear, the woman would get out the childbed linen she had set aside, and make up her bed for the travail. While the contractions were still mild and far apart, she would probably continue with her chores or, as some midwifery manuals recommended, walk around the house. When the labor pains increased in intensity, and it became clear that this was no false alarm but true travail, she would send her husband for the midwife and the neighbors.

After arriving, the midwife might build up the fire if the day was cold, or set up her birthing stool if she had one. Men and children would be shooed from the room, and the neighbors and midwife would make provisions for privacy. In many households this would probably be, at best, a set of curtains drawn closely around the bed; in other, wealthier, families a separate room was set aside. The midwife would lubricate her hands with butter, almond oil, or lard, and perform an internal examination to check the woman's cervical dilation. Once she had done that, the midwife could announce how long a wait it would be.

Until the waters broke, the midwife and her assistants would encourage the woman in labor to walk around the room. If she seemed weak, one of the attendants might prepare some broth or boil some eggs—the same foods recommended for invalids. Mostly, all the assembled women could do was wait. Now was the time for the exchange of gossip and news—or for comparing stories of past travails. Unless the mother-to-be was in unusual pain, this was likely a cheerful and celebratory time, with the conversation peppered with jokes and bawdy stories.

If things began to go wrong, a good midwife had some skills at her disposal. Many midwives knew how to turn the child in the womb, preferably so that it would be born "naturally"—that is, head first. In other cases, it was necessary to turn the child feet first. Midwives and laywomen alike had medicinal recipes at their disposal to give strength to the mother and to hasten labor. Many of these recipes contained pennyroyal, rue, juniper, and other herbs associated with "female complaints." Some might well have had the effect of encouraging uterine contractions, as might the practice of having the woman drink another woman's milk.

When the woman's contractions increased, and grew to the second, or pushing, stage of labor, two or more of the assembled women would assist the mother to the birth stool or the edge of the bed. Two women would hold her under the arms; others might support her back or hold her legs. The midwife would position herself to catch the child as it emerged. The midwife or another woman might coat her hands with oil or butter and massage the woman's stomach with each contraction; or the midwife might lubricate the birth canal with goose grease or almond oil. The midwife would encourage the woman to hold her breath and bear down.

After the child was born, the midwife would cut the umbilical cord and bind the stump with a cloth belly band. While she attended to delivering the afterbirth, another woman would bathe the child (in warm wine if possible), swaddle it, and put it in the waiting cradle. Since it was believed that colostrum (the fluid in women's breasts that precedes true milk) was bad for the child, another woman would suckle it or feed it barley water or gruel. The midwife, meanwhile, would swaddle the mother's thighs and belly with some of the linen the mother had put aside for this purpose. This swaddling prevented cold air from entering the womb and inciting a childbed fever. If she was still in pain from postpartum contractions, one of the neighbors might give her a cordial or drink to soothe these so-called afterpains. Any bloody or stained cloth would be taken away to be washed, and the mother would be officially "put to bed," where she would lie in for two weeks to a month. One of the neighbor women, a teenage girl, or a paid nurse would stay with her to help with the household chores and to attend to her other needs. The other women would disperse, perhaps returning in a day or two for a celebratory postpartum meal.

AREAS OF AMBIGUITY

Housewives and midwives tended their families and neighbors without undue suspicion or interference. However, there were two areas where women's medical practice balanced on the border of legitimate and illegitimate practice: the prescription and use of abortifacients, and the use of healing magic. While both practices were acceptable under some circumstances, they were not under others.

Research on abortion in colonial America is scant. Many scholars of this period stress that sexuality was so closely connected with reproduction that abortion and birth control were rare to the point of nonexistence. Recently, however, a few historians have begun to suggest that abortion may have been much more common than previously thought, especially among unmarried women. Some evidence even suggests that abortion was a common form of birth control among German women in eighteenth-century Philadelphia.[31]

Included in the Brigham women's recipes for female complaints are two concoctions that seem to be intended to induce abortion. Both examples are ambiguous; neither recipe explicitly uses the word *abortion*. However, internal evidence, especially in the second example, strongly suggests that at least one of these potions was in fact an abortifacient. These recipes tend to support the contention that early American women did practice abortion, although with some qualification.

Consider the two Brigham recipes. A prescription to "heale any outward or inward wounde" includes the warning, "Let no woman wth childe drink this for it will help to doe ye office of a midwife."[32] The context is not clear enough to determine whether this is a sincere warning or a code phrase indicating that the medicine would induce a miscarriage. According to a modern herbal, the ingredients in this recipe are generally vasoconstrictors and styptics, herbs that would help to stop bleeding. There is no evidence that the herbs had secondary uses as abortifacients.[33]

The second recipe is more problematic. It is called, "To cleanse the Womb":

> Take maddeer roots, Juniper berries; Bayberries, corriander seeds of each an ounce, Currance halfe a pound; mother time, mother wort, muggwort, sanicle, of each a large handfull; bruise all well, & boyle ym in a gallon of beere till a quart be waisted, then put in a quart of white wine, . . . then take it offe & straine it out & put it up into bottles, & drinke of it constantly halfe a pinte in ye morning first, & last at night goeing to bed at the last four days before you have them and all the time you have them; when you see they are come, put in halfe a drame of saffron powdered into a draught & drinke it offe. It will be least offensive to drink it pretty hot.[34]

Of the herbs listed in this recipe, six are known abortifacients: madder roots, juniper berries, mother-of-thyme, mugwort, motherwort, and saffron. Most notable is the use of juniper, which may have referred to the infamous abortifacient called savin, a species of juniper.[35]

The question remains, however, whether the women who used these recipes were consciously inducing abortion or not. In the humoral medicine paradigm, "suppressed" or "obstructed" menses was a recognized malady. Menstruation was nature's way of purging poisonous humors from a woman's body. If they remained, the putrefying humors could make the woman sick.[36] If a young woman's period was late, she might ask her mother or aunt for a drink to bring it on, without knowing—or admitting—she was pregnant. One mid-

"To Cleanse the Womb," a recipe from the Brigham family medical recipe book. This recipe includes ingredients that might induce abortion. (Courtesy, American Antiquarian Society.)

wifery manual acknowledged that this sometimes happened—interestingly enough, blaming male physicians when it did:

> For, when after conception a woman finds an Alteration in herself, and yet knows not from whence it arises, she is apt to run to a Doctor, and enquire of him what the Matter is, who, not knowing she is with Child, gives her perhaps a strong cathartical poison, which certainly will destroy the conception.[37]

It seems likely that the real use of these recipes lay somewhere between a conscious desire for abortion and a naive belief in obstructed menses. Since there was no way to confirm a pregnancy before "quickening," or fetal movement, women could use these recipes to rid themselves of possible pregnancies before they knew for sure they were with child. Thus, these recipes were and were not true abortifacients. Language in the recipe is further evidence of the ambiguity of its purpose. The user is instructed to add saffron when "you see they are come." The word *they* probably refers to the "terms," a common way of referring to menstruation. Women using this medicine may well have thought of it as a way of inducing menstruation, not abortion, whatever the real effects may have been.

The Brigham women were not alone in their ambivalence. The legal status of abortion in the seventeenth century made early pregnancy terminations an area of undefined legal consequences for women. The first English statute on abortion, promulgated in 1623, defines criminal abortion as one that takes place after quickening.[38] Early references in American court records are ambiguous at best. One 1677 case from Groton, Massachusetts, makes veiled references to a young woman's crime that could signify either criminal abortion or infanticide. Hannah Blood had run away from the household where she had been a servant. Before she disappeared, she had been seen to be "big as a woman with child useth to be," but she would not admit to being pregnant. When she was last seen, her "great belly" had disappeared, and a visitor "saw her lying on ye bed for her cariage and demeanor of herselfe as woman in yt condition," that is, a woman newly delivered of a child. The court wanted to find Blood because she was "supposed to have had a child, and in a wicked manner hath ben made away." Significantly, one witness testified that she had seen Hannah Blood taking savin. From the evidence that was recorded, it is not clear whether the court's interest in Blood's whereabouts stemmed from suspicion of infanticide, abortion, or merely running away from her master. What is clear is that she probably had been pregnant, that she had been seen taking an abortifacient, and that there was no sign of an infant.[39]

There were no American prosecutions explicitly for abortion until the 1740s. In one of the earliest cases, a doctor was prosecuted, not for obliterating the fetus but for the death of the mother in the course of "destroying the fruit of her womb." In this case, it was the physician who was prosecuted, and then only for performing a late-term abortion, after quickening. Overall, the evidence on abortion in early America seems to indicate that any stigma associated with terminating a pregnancy stemmed not from the killing of a fetus but from the illicit sex that created it: "abortion was understood as blameworthy because it was an extreme action designed to hide a prior sin, sex outside of marriage."[40]

For all women, then, the ambiguity of early pregnancy created an opportunity to control fertility and, for single women, a way to escape the consequences of a fornication charge. How conscious each woman was of terminating a pregnancy when she used recipes like those of the Brighams probably varied from one woman to another. They passed the recipes among themselves just as they did those to prevent miscarriage and increase the flow of breast milk, but perhaps they were conveyed with a whisper and accompanied by a significant look. It seems likely that the purpose of medicines like this one remained understood but unspoken.

The use of supernatural interventions in healing was another area of ambiguity and unspoken understandings. In the worldview of a religious Puritan, prayer, fasting, and other rituals designed to invoke the supernatural were as much a part of healing as cordials and possets. Sickness had two causes: imbalanced humors were the physical cause, and sin was the spiritual cause. The sin could be the patient's own or that of a loved one. Indeed, many parents spent time atoning for their own sins when their children were sick.[41] Early Americans also used more direct means of manipulating supernatural power, means that we would call magic or spells. Some practiced divination to locate lost objects, animals, or even people. Others used magic to protect themselves from witches or discover thieves or vandals. Healing spells were also widespread and included a wide variety of practices. Despite attempts by the clergy to eliminate them, in the popular mind such practices were not incompatible with Christian piety. Most laypeople were eclectic in their spiritual practices. Religion and prayer answered some needs; magic and charms, others. They played different roles in everyday life and thus did not come into direct conflict with each other. Ordinary people kept the two practices separate in their minds as well. "Most layfolk who practiced magic seem to have lacked . . . intellectual self-consciousness," when it came to the relationship between magic and religion.[42]

With this background, one can begin to interpret the ambiguous and sometimes bizarre recipes that turn up so often in the records of both male and female practitioners. Dr. Talman of Guilford, Connecticut, copied into his commonplace book a recipe to cure deafness that begins as follows: "Take a Bate [bat] and Clean hem Leave his head on hes Eyes in, his Skin on and hang him up by the head." The recipe continues with instructions for extracting oil from the bat and applying it to the patient's ears with "neger's wool."[43] Talman made no explicit mention of magic in this prescription, but the oddity of using a bat and the instructions to use a specific kind of human hair suggest that the recipe took at least part of its efficacy from the supernatural.

In many recipes, what now seem to be bizarre ingredients and magical ritual originated in contemporary science. Massachusetts physician John Barton recorded instructions "to cure a green wound by the weapon that gave it," which involved applying an ointment to the weapon instead of the patient. The ointment itself contained such ingredients as "moss growing upon a scull" and "oyl of snails."[44] This particular prescription is a variation on the famous "weapon salve" of Sir Kenelm Digby, who claimed that his salve would cause a patient's "vital spirits" and lost blood to leave the weapon and return to the patient. Digby explicitly stated that this cure was based completely on natural forces and made no use of magic or the occult. Despite Digby's disclaimer, it is not clear that all who used this method thought of it as a nonmagical cure. In the popular mind, "it is doubtful that this use of sympathetic cures was justified on this rarefied intellectual basis."[45] Thus, for some practitioners, this was a physical cure; for others, a magical one.

Even such clerics as Cotton Mather sometimes resorted to the supernatural when there was sickness in their families. When Mather's first wife was dying of breast cancer, she dreamed that a mysterious "grave person" suggested that she apply warm wool "from a living sheep" to her breast. Their physician "mightily encouraged our trying the Experiments."[46] The physician saw merit in the method, despite its origin. Both of the Mathers attributed the apparition to divine intervention—not, as one might expect, to Satanic influences.[47]

It is not surprising, then, that women practitioners also used healing magic. A female relative brought scarlet cloth with her when she visited the Sewalls after the birth of their first child. She suggested that the new parents lay the cloth on the child's head to protect it from sickness.[48] The Brighams included many recipes and instructions that had magical elements. The notebook records several recipes for a strange concoction called "swallow water," which is not unlike the bat recipe transcribed by Dr. Talman:

> Take 40 or 50 young swallowes wn they be ready to fly out of their nests ye more ye better, bruiseing ym feathers & all in a morter to paste, add to ym 2 ounces of castoreum beaten into fine powder, & 3 pintes of strong white wine viniger, mix all thise well together & sett it in a still & distill it as rose water.[49]

Swallows were important birds in English folklore. Some believed that it was dangerous, even fatal to harm a swallow or disturb its nest;

clearly the Brighams followed a different tradition. At any rate, swallows had powers beyond the natural, powers that the Brighams called on when they used this recipe. The medicine would cure just about anything that ailed man or beast, including heart disease and apoplexy.[50]

Birds turn up again in the Brighams' instructions for nursing a person through the plague:

> For swelling under ye Eares, Armepitts, or in ye groines, draw
> them forth & breake ym wth all speed thus: Pull offe ye feathers from offe ye tayles of liveing cocks, Hens, Pidgions, or
> chickens, & holding their bills fast, hold them hard to ye botch
> or swelling & so keepe yem at ye parte until they dye.[51]

This practice was a common form of English healing magic in which the disease was "transferred" to an animal.[52] The Brighams also used astrology in their prescriptions. Most of these uses of astrology were of the kind discussed earlier, recommendations for propitious days for planting or gathering medicinal plants. For example, one recipe directs the user as follows: "The Pyony roote is taken up wn ye Lune is in Leo, & upon Sunday before ye full of ye moone."[53] However, the Brighams did not rely on astrology as much as other practitioners. Some doctors in England practiced entirely by astrological chart without even needing to see a patient.[54]

Despite the widespread use of magic in healing, it was possible to cross the line from acceptable practice to criminal intent. The following 1680 witchcraft case from Hampton, New Hampshire, demonstrates the danger of pushing magical healing too far. One woman's healing methods frightened her neighbors so badly that they had her arrested for witchcraft.

When the toddler Moses Godfrey fell sick, the Godfreys' neighbor Rachel Fuller came to offer her help. She patted the child's hand and assured Goodwife Godfrey that "the child will be well." What she did next, however, confirmed the latent suspicions of the Godfreys that Rachel Fuller was a witch. First, Fuller daubed her face and hands with molasses, then "the said Rachel Fuller turned her about, and smote the back of her hands together sundry times, and spat in the fire. Then she, having herbs in her hands, stood and rubbed them in her hand and strewed them about the hearth by the fire." Fuller left soon thereafter, but Goodwife Godfrey and her daughter Sarah observed the following outside their house: they "saw Rachel Fuller standing with her face toward the house, and beat herself with her arms, as men do in winter to heat their hands, and this she did three times; and stooping down and gathering something off the ground in the interim between the beating of herself, and then she went home."[55]

It did not help Fuller's case that the Godfreys were already suspicious of her before the incident with the sick child occurred. Indeed, she had brought much of this suspicion on herself, by claiming to know of many witches practicing in Hampton and by giving unsolicited advice on how to guard against witchcraft and spells. Such intimate knowledge of witches and witchcraft could only come from one who was herself a witch. The Godfreys tried to keep Fuller away from their house, and when she came in and took the sick child's hand again, Goodwife Godfrey snatched his hand away and wrapped it in her apron.[56]

Since Rachel Fuller's reputation as a witch had preceded her, it colored the Godfreys' interpretation of her behavior. However, this was no ordinary healing. Fuller's use of magic had overstepped the bounds of acceptable practice. The Brighams' magical recipes were close enough to ordinary medicines to pass muster, even if they contained strange ingredients like live birds. Such recipes balanced on the line between the natural and the magical, with no explicit invocation of supernatural forces. Rachel Fuller's behavior—smearing molasses on her face, performing an odd little dance outside the Godfreys' house—could easily be interpreted as calling on Satan or spirits to assist her healing. The Godfreys apparently thought so. When Moses died of his illness, they had Fuller arrested for witchcraft and murder.

Some writers have used cases like Fuller's to argue that women healers were particularly vulnerable to witchcraft accusations. These writers contend that the male medical profession deliberately targeted midwives and other female practitioners in order to wipe out competition. Yet many—indeed the majority—of women healers practiced without harassment in both England and America. These same healers incorporated magical elements into their activities as a matter of course—again, without harassment or even much comment. While there is an association between healing and witchcraft, this association is more complex than it first seems.[57]

Medical practice was just one female activity among many that could be perverted to Satan's purposes. A study of witchcraft in England points out that women's work—spinning, churning, brewing, and dairying—was particularly susceptible to supernatural interference. American cases demonstrate a similar pattern. It seems that part of the association between healers and witchcraft stems not from healing per se, but from its association with women. Since women were thought to be more likely to become witches in the first place, any deviation from normal practices in their work—whether healing, brewing, or baking—could find them accused. Healing activity was associated with witchcraft accusations in most cases because it was women's work. Rachel Fuller ended up an accused witch not just because she was a healer, but for a combination of factors: her magical practices overstepped the bounds of the acceptable; she already had a reputation as a witch; and perhaps most important, her healing failed spectacularly. There is, however, one set of circumstances under which healers were more vulnerable than other women: when women practiced independently and for money. For the average housewife, however, healing was no more dangerous than any other kind of work.[58]

At the core of all parts of household practice is the fact that most everyday care of the sick was the domain of women. Like knowledge of brewing and baking, healing skills were passed on from mother to daughter as part of household management. Midwives and doctoresses parlayed their medical knowledge into paid work and community service. Such skills took them (and some particularly skilled housewives) into a variety of contexts, from the homes of the poor to the halls of the courthouse.

No one, male or female, had a monopoly on medical practice. At times, women healers worked cooperatively with men; at other times, they ignored male healers; and at still other times, they challenged male physicians as direct competitors. In all of these contexts, medical skills gave women a certain measure of autonomy and authority, themes that will come up again and again as we explore the extent of women's practice. Yet women's practice had limits as well. Some limits were inherent in the definition of female practice; others were imposed from the outside and enforced with social sanctions. All forms of women's practice, however, began and centered on the household, the housewife, and the bedside of sick family members.

[3]

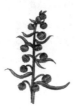

Calling the Women
Medical Networks and Women's Communities

IN THE FRIGID PREDAWN of December 26, 1738, Hannah Parkman went into labor. Her husband Ebenezer got out of bed, saddled his horse, and rode for the midwife, Granny Forbush. After he left Mrs. Forbush in the bedchamber with his wife, he went back into the cold to collect his first wife's sister, Mrs. Hicks; neighbors Mrs. Knowlton, Mrs. Whipple, Mrs. Byles, and Mrs. Rogers; and the doctoress Hepzibah Maynard, also a neighbor. The women stayed all day and into the evening, when Mrs. Parkman's contractions stopped. Mrs. Forbush sent everyone home, but she stayed with her patient. At dawn on December 28, Mrs. Forbush came out of the bedchamber and awakened Ebenezer. Mrs. Parkman was in labor again, and the birth appeared imminent; "with great earnestness," she asked Ebenezer to gather the women again. Ebenezer once again rushed into the night to reassemble his wife's attendants. Three hours later, after a short but very painful labor, Mrs. Parkman, surrounded by her sister-in-law, five female neighbors, and the midwife, gave birth to the Parkmans' fourth daughter. Ebenezer, who had been waiting outside the bedchamber, received the news from Granny Forbush.[1]

Such scenes were commonplace in early America and would remain so well into the nineteenth century. Gathering groups of women to attend others in childbirth or sickness was so common, in fact, that it is possible to overlook its significance. Why gather large groups of women to attend others, when a midwife and one or two attendants could perform the actual medical tasks perfectly well? The answer is that women's medical gatherings had social as well as practical functions. Medical care as part of a woman's calling had consequences that reached beyond the individual household and into the community as a whole. The loose groups of neighbors that characterized women's household doctoring coalesced into clusters, communities of women. These communities—some transient, some persistent—were centered around medical care and practice. Membership focused on shared physical experience, especially childbirth. Women began their initiation into such groups as teenagers, when they took turns watching at bedsides and running errands for new mothers, and became adult participants when they gave birth to their first child.

Medical gatherings filled a special function for women. They were a place where women met with each other for shared work, celebration, mourning, and talk. Such gatherings were important parts of seventeenth-century public life. There were two kinds of "publics" in the seventeenth century. One was involved in institutional structures like churches and governments; another, equally important public consisted of groups of peers who "saw each other frequently and commented on each other's doings." The judgments and sanctions of the informal, peer-based public could be even more important in an individual's life than the distant decisions of the formal, institutional public.[2]

Medical gatherings were an especially important subset of the informal public for women. They served a number of supportive functions, starting with medical care and extending into other kinds of services and material support. Women's medical networks were also important to larger social structures and institutions, as when women's sickbed networks served to bind families and factions together. Under other circumstances, the women's medical communities created a power base from which to pursue their own interests in community disputes. However, as both a social structure and a public forum, the bonds women formed with each other at sickbeds and childbirths were double-edged. Medical gatherings could be sources of empowerment, yet they could also be sources of bitter and persistent quarrels.

THE STRUCTURE OF WOMEN'S COMMUNITIES

The origins of women's medical communities lie in the social clusterings that surrounded the sick and women in labor. Social medicine, as it has been called, entailed both sociability and medical practice. Childbirth practices were particularly congenial to the development of women's communities, and that atmosphere remained remarkably consistent over time.[3] During the colonial period, men were always excluded from attendance at normal births. Indeed, "calling the women" defined the beginning of active labor. Every pregnant woman, wealthy or poor, respectable matron or unmarried servant, expected to be surrounded by a group of women when her time came. Circumstances that prevented this from happening were a cause of distress. Samuel Sewall of Boston wrote in his diary for 1690:

> Tuesday, August 12. . . .Note: My wife was so ill could hardly
> get home, taking some harm in going in Pattens, or some
> wrench, so had a great flux of Blood, which amaz'd us both, at
> last my wife bad me call Mrs. Ellis, then, Mother Hull, then
> the Midwife, and throw the Goodness of God was brought to
> Bed of a Daughter between 3. and four aclock, August 13th
> 1690. . . . Mrs. Elisabeth Weeden, Midwife. Had not Women
> nor other preparations, as usually, being wholly surpris'd, my
> wife expecting to have gone a Moneth longer.[4]

Mrs. Sewall was not alone for her precipitous birth; she was attended by her mother and two midwives. Yet her husband commented that she "had not women." Clearly the expectation was that there would be a much larger group, if they had only had the time to make the proper "preparations." Similarly, Cotton Mather found it worth noting in 1709 that his wife gave birth very quickly, before there was time to send for more than one or two neighbors.[5]

Contemporary midwifery manuals described a group of "good women" as a medical as well as a social necessity. The anonymous author of *Aristotle's Compleat Masterpiece* prescribed "a Pallet-Bed girded and placed near the Fire, that the good Women may come on each Side," as the best arrangement for delivery. If labor proceeded slowly, "let a woman hold her two Shoulders, that she may strain out the Birth with the more Advantage."[6] Gathering the neighboring women was as important as calling the midwife.

Every woman expected a large group of neighbors and relatives when she gave birth, and she had an equal obligation to attend others. Shortly after the events described at the beginning of this chapter, Ebenezer Parkman had to fend off the complaints of a woman who was "disgusted" that he had prevented Mrs. Parkman from attending her previous lying-in. (Interestingly, Parkman made the excuse that he himself had been ill that day, and his wife had to tend to him.)[7]

There was also a ceremonial aspect to childbirth. Distinctive foods and ritual visiting set lying-in apart not just from ordinary life but from other kinds of illnesses as well. Samuel Sewall brewed a special "groaning beer" for his wife shortly before the birth of their first child; he later recorded (with evident relish) the menus of the meals his wife shared with her attendants: "Women din'd with Rost Beef and minc'd Pyes, good cheese and Tarts," he wrote in 1694. After the birth of their last child, Mrs. Sewall felt even more celebratory, as Mr. Sewall noted: "My wife treats her midwife and women: Had a good Dinner, Boil'd Pork, Beef, Fowls: very good Rost Beef; Turkey Pye, Tarts." Sixteen women attended this feast.[8] Women such as Mary Holyoke continued these celebrations for an entire week. After each of her births, Mrs. Holyoke chose a week to be her "sitting up week," during which she received many visitors. She also made note of other women's sitting up weeks and paid visits herself, to drink tea and see the new baby.[9] Such elaborate rituals may have been the province of well-off women such as Mrs. Sewall and Mrs. Holyoke, but their poorer counterparts also attended their neighbors, even if there were no delicacies to eat or tea to drink.

What binds all of these events together is the all-female guest list. Mr. Sewall was not invited to share the roast beef and turkey pies; Dr. Holyoke was conspicuously absent from the visits to sitting up women. Not only was the birth itself women's province, but so was the social time that came afterward. Here was one place where women's fertility was acknowledged and (as in the case of Mrs. Sewall) celebrated. This celebration depended on the common experience of pregnancy and childbirth. Only married women appear on the lists of guests at births, and while it is not explicitly stated, they probably also were all mothers. Women freely commented on each other's reproductive status. When Mary Drury of Boston complained to Rachel Harwood in 1677 that she was not well, Harwood replied, "I did think she was with child." Drury dismissed this assumption, but Harwood insisted that she could tell when a woman was pregnant, and assured Drury that she was "not so old but that she might have children."[10] Women also empathized with each other's pain during labor. When one woman badgered another about the possible illegitimacy of her child, another attendant rebuked the questioner, saying, "Leave her alone . . . she has trouble enough now."[11]

Though the women-centered nature of childbirth attendance is a commonplace of early American life, groups of women gathered at bedsides in a similar way for almost any illness or injury. A good housewife nursed her family through illnesses. Sickness in the family also brought other women to the bedside, including neighbors and kin. The female exclusivity was not as strict as at childbirth, especially if the patient was male. Still, care for the sick was undoubtedly a female province.

When John Davenport Jr. was ill in 1666, his father and his parents' manservant Edmund participated in his care. They, like his mother Elizabeth, sat at his bedside as watchers, keeping an eye on his condition, but his mother and her female neighbors were clearly in charge of his care. When John Jr. became so weak that he could not turn over in bed by himself, John Sr. noted that it took two women to lift him. It was Mrs. Bache and Mrs. Fairechild who brought medicines to try and whose advice was taken seriously. Elizabeth was willing to try Mrs. Bache's "water made with minte and sack and saunders distilled, with a little bagg of ambergreece hangd in it," although she was more dubious of Mrs. Fairechild's concoction made of sheep guts. However, when Nicholas Auger, a physician, recommended cinquefoil steeped in white wine, she treated his recommendation as an afterthought.[12]

Other male diarists and letter writers made note of the crowds of women around every sickbed. William Leete wrote to the physician John Winthrop Jr. in great distress when his infant daughter developed an illness "such as none of our woemen can tell that they have ever seen the like."[13] Ebenezer Parkman took a different attitude when his wife was sick in 1739. So many women were in the house that he found it "an unspeakable hindrance to my studies."[14]

People of the time saw differences between sickbeds and childbirths. Childbirth was not yet the pathologized event it was to become in the late eighteenth century, and was not cause for medical intervention such as the use of forceps. Childbirth, unlike illness, was a happy occasion, as Mrs. Sewall's feasts indicate. But there were also considerable similarities. Both childbirth and illness were occasions for fear. Any illness was potentially fatal in an age before accurate diagnosis or effective drugs. Women about to give birth settled their affairs and made their peace with God. Cotton Mather wrote in a 1724 essay aimed at pregnant women, "your Death has entered into you."[15] Women did die in childbirth regularly enough to make this a not unreasonable perception. Attendants on both the sick and the parturient provided medicines, soothing drinks, and poultices to their charges in an effort to make them more comfortable and stave off complications.

The two events—illness and childbirth—were also similar to other forms of female sociability. In a sense, medical gatherings were merely another place where women assembled to work together. Just as women gathered at a sickbed or a birth, they often met each other at a community well or cow pen, where they drew water or milked together. At other times, women joined each other to spin or to help with the harvest. While they worked, they also talked—just as they did while tending the sick.[16]

Medical gatherings also shared certain characteristics with women's religious gatherings. So-called private meetings for prayer and Bible study were an important part of several Protestant sects in New England, including both the Puritans and the Quakers. Some of these groups were mixtures of men and women, but many involved only one gender. As the Puritan church became more of a female domain during the seventeenth century, these women's meetings became more and more popular. Most often, they were led by women, although it was not unusual for a women's prayer group to invite a male minister to speak to them. Like medical groups, prayer gatherings brought women together in an intimate setting, for a common purpose, and they allowed women to take positions of leadership that were usually reserved for men.[17]

In all of these groups, women could be alone with each other and could participate in a set of social relationships and obligations that excluded men. Prayer groups, work groups, and medical groups often overlapped, in both social and functional terms: a prayer group might gather at a sick member's bedside, or a woman in labor might ask that women who shared her cow pen be called to the birth. But medical gatherings were especially conducive to the formation of women's social networks, since they emphasized the mutual dependency of those gathered. Indeed, the material function of the groups was to create a pool of communal skills that could be depended on to save a life or at least reduce suffering. Perhaps most important, sickbeds involved hours and hours of waiting, watching, and talking. These bedside conversations ensured that those who engaged in them knew a great deal of each others' business, whether they wanted to or not.

Such intimacy could have two contrasting outcomes: warm affection or bitter rivalry. The story of the Parkman women and their neighbors provides a vivid example of the centrality of medical practice in women's social networks, and of how (in this case) the intimacy of the bedside led to lifelong bonds between families. Both of Ebenezer Parkman's wives became part of medically based women's networks when they gave birth to their first infants. As time passed, the relationships that began in the birth chamber developed and grew. In fact, in many ways the women who first came to attend births took on many of the duties of kin.

Kin served a number of functions in early America. Demographic studies indicate that early New Englanders were particularly likely to live close to family members and to have "intense" relationships with their relatives in the immediate geographic area. As a result, family and community were deeply intertwined. One's neighbors were often one's relatives, and one's relatives were often one's neighbors. Communities took a deep interest in families and family relationships. Neighbors as well as kin gave their opinions on potential marriages, child-rearing practices, and family quarrels.[18]

Extended families had high expectations for each other. Claiming a distant kin relationship was a way of extracting favors from a higher-placed person. One historian described the tone of such requests as mixing "hyperbole and obsequiousness." Nevertheless, such requests usually generated a positive response. Extended kin relationships, however tenuous, carried weight with the Anglo-Americans of the seventeenth century. Indeed, such ties were maintained in some families even across the ocean, and kin in subsequent generations kept up the connection, even though they had never laid eyes on one another. Such ties served purposes beyond the sentimental. For male family members, extended kin networks often developed into "preferential trading relationships" that served to benefit all parties.[19]

Women's medical networks demonstrate the importance of female kin. Kin networks, whether literal or fictive, guaranteed appropriate medical care during childbirth and family illnesses. They provided a pool of female medical skills on which the nuclear family could draw when the skills of the housewife were not enough. As these networks became more established and elaborate, they gave rise to other kin-like obligations and behavior.

In some cases, the kinship tie had a shaky basis in fact. For instance, after Ebenezer Parkman's first wife, Molly Champney Parkman, died in 1736, her kin fully adopted his second wife, Hannah Breck Parkman, into their family. Rebecca Champney Hicks, Molly's sister, maintained her contact with her brother-in-law and was at Hannah's bedside when she miscarried her first pregnancy in February 1738. Hannah had no living sisters of her own; Rebecca Hicks played the part of a sister for her. In the end, Rebecca attended more of Hannah's deliveries than she did of Molly's. Rebecca truly became "Sister Hicks" to Hannah Parkman, despite the lack of literal blood ties.[20]

Rebecca Hicks not only treated Hannah Parkman like blood kin but also drew Hannah into the Champney kin network. In December 1738, Parkman suffered through three days of labor that left her very weak and the baby sickly. Hicks sent her own daughter, Ruth, to "watch" with Parkman, who was so feeble she could not stand upright without fainting. After the infant died, Parkman's condition worsened; she was still unable to walk on her own, and her "lower Limbs [grew] useless and one of her feet swells." Rebecca Hicks and her daughter were two of the "divers women" who came to the Parkman house during this crisis; in addition, Hicks recruited her cousin, Elizabeth Champney Winchester, to come and nurse Parkman. Through her marriage, Hannah acquired not just a set of Parkman in-laws, but another set of Champney kin through Ebenezer's first wife. This set of "adopted" kin grew out of women's business of healing— primarily childbirth, but not entirely. Rebecca Hicks helped nurse Hannah and the Parkman children through an outbreak of measles, tended Hannah after she was thrown by a horse, and sent both Ruth and her other daughter Bekky to tend Ebenezer when he was ill.[21]

This process was not limited to women who could claim some kind of kin connection, however tenuous. Childbirth and sickbed gatherings brought together women related only by physical proximity, yet these coincidental connections developed into networks of "fictive kin" as elaborate as blood ties. Both Hannah and Molly Parkman entered into the kin networks of neighboring women in this fashion. Two Westborough families in particular, the Forbushes and the Maynards, took the Parkman women into their circles. At first, these families were chosen because they lived close by; when they first visited the Parkman home, Ebenezer described them merely as neighbors. As time passed, however, the relationship became much more complex and intimate. The neighboring women began bringing their own sisters, daughters, and daughters-in-law to the Parkmans, and some of these women began to attend not just to Hannah and Molly but to Ebenezer and the children as well.

Dorcas "Granny" Forbush was the local midwife. She delivered at least eight of the sixteen Parkman children, and saw Hannah through a miscarriage and a stillbirth as well. At first, she attended the Parkman women on her own, accepting the assistance of other neighbors and Molly's and Hannah's kin. As time went on, however, she began to bring her own female relations with her to Hannah Parkman's deliveries, including her daughter-in-law Susanna, her sister-in-law Sarah Forbush, and even her granddaughter-in-law.[22]

The Maynard women also had a tradition of medical care that was passed down through the generations. Of the Maynard women mentioned in the Parkman diary, two practiced as unpaid doctoresses, offering highly skilled, non-childbirth-related care. One eventually replaced Granny Forbush as the community's midwife after Forbush's death. David Maynard Sr. and his wife were originally the Parkmans' landlords, but through the women's medical network, a complex relationship developed between the two extended families. "Madam" Maynard, wife of David Sr., the landowner, attended many of the Parkman women in labor. Her name first appears in the diary as one of Molly's watchers in 1726, when Molly suffered serious complications after the birth of her first child. She soon began to involve her large family in her relationship with the Parkmans. When Hannah Parkman's first pregnancy ended in a late-term miscarriage, David and Madam's teenage son, Ebenezer, dug a grave for the dead infant. When Hannah fell ill in 1746, Madam Maynard took the youngest Parkman infant and asked her daughter-in-law to suckle her until Hannah recovered. Like Granny Forbush, Madam Maynard also brought her female kin with her when she attended the Parkman women in labor, including her nieces, her daughters-in-law, and most importantly, her sister-in-law Hepzibah.[23]

Hepzibah Maynard was a doctoress with an extensive practice. She was born Hepzibah Brigham, a member of the same Brigham family that passed down the medical recipe book discussed in the previous chapter. She first attended one of Hannah Parkman's births in 1738, but soon began to attend the Parkman family under other circumstances as well. When Billy Parkman nearly severed his foot with an ax in 1750, Ebenezer sent for her before anyone else. She nursed Ebenezer during a serious illness in 1752.[24] Hepzibah also served as "second in command" at childbeds and may have acted as chief midwife when Granny Forbush was unavailable. The Parkmans' relationship with Hepzibah Maynard eventually stretched beyond the female world of healing and into other areas. Ebenezer appears to have been quite fond of her and was very pleased to report that she came to dinner at the Parkman house in 1757 "after many entreaties." When she died later that year, Parkman honored her by choosing for her funeral sermon the Proverbs text "Who can find a virtuous woman? For her price is far above rubies."[25] After many years of friendship, the Parkman and Maynard families were finally united when Hannah's niece married Hepzibah's son Stephen in 1759.[26]

Once the ties were established, both the Forbushes and the Maynards treated the Parkmans as intimates. Granny Forbush was a frequent dinner guest at the Parkmans, and Ebenezer and Hannah appeared at the Forbushes' table just as often. Sometimes Mrs. Forbush brought the Parkmans gifts, as on April 6, 1747, when she appeared at their door with a peck and a half of "excellent Flax seed."[27] The Maynards were even more generous. Hepzibah Maynard's grandson came by the Parkman house in January 1756 with a gift of beef and suet from his grandfather. He also brought a gift of black cloth for Ebenezer's winter coat. The Parkmans reciprocated such favors. Two years later, Ebenezer made a gift of a devotional book to Hepzibah's sister, Mary.[28]

These exchanges of goods were more than tokens of affection. In an economy with little cash, both formal and informal barter was essential. Without the exchanges made possible by the Parkman women's social and medical network, the Parkmans and Maynards would have been hard-pressed to provide food, clothing, and medicine for their rapidly expanding families. Many of the goods traded were products of women's domestic labor: cloth, preserved and otherwise processed food, garden seeds, and medicine. What appear at first to be gifts may well have been the settling of accounts between the women of the two families. The women kept no account books but remembered who owed whom, right to the last flax seed or yard of cloth. When Ebenezer got involved in the exchange, it was to offer a resource to which he had more access than his wife: a printed book. In this way, women's networks connected them not just to the local economy but also to manufactured goods and the transatlantic trade, as exemplified by Ebenezer's "gift."[29]

Harmonious and affectionate relationships like those between the Parkman and Maynard families were one result of sickbed intimacy, but other kinds of relationships also grew there. The intense relationships that developed between women at sickbeds and childbirths had the potential to explode into equally intense conflicts. Familiarity bred contempt as easily as love, and when it did, there were serious consequences for the women involved. If emotions ran high enough, what began as a squabble at a sickbed could escalate to accusations of witchcraft—what one historian called the "seventeenth-century verbal equivalents of nuclear weapons."[30] The gossip that characterized women's medical gatherings demonstrates that the women's medical community had the ability to destroy a reputation and a life as well as save one.

The little-known Hartford witch-hunt is a case in point. It was the only "panic" witch-hunt in America other than the one in Salem, and its relative obscurity stems, no doubt, from the sparse documentation that survives. However, from the remaining evidence, it is clear that the women's medical networks played an important role in initiating and escalating the hunt.

The immediate background to the Hartford witch-hunt was a religious dispute known as the "Hartford Controversy." While there is a "lamentable lack of hard detail" about the dispute, it seems likely that it concerned the religious doctrine of the "halfway covenant," a proposal to loosen the criteria for baptism. At about the same time, there was a severe epidemic with a high mortality rate. Shortly after these tensions gripped the community, the witch-hunt began.[31]

The first accusations stemmed from incidents at a sickbed—that of an eight-year-old girl, Elizabeth Kelly. The chain of events that culminated in witchcraft accusations began innocuously enough. Goodwife Ayres stopped by the Kellys' house one Sunday morning. While there, she helped herself to some broth "hot out of the boiling pot" that hung on the hearth. She then called to young Elizabeth and offered her some of the broth. The adult Kellys warned their daughter that the broth was too hot for her, but the child drank some anyway. Almost immediately, Elizabeth began to complain of pains in her belly.[32]

At first, Bethia Kelly, Elizabeth's mother, didn't think much of it. Children were always having stomach aches, and hadn't she warned Elizabeth that the soup was too hot? Goodwife Kelly gave her daughter a dose of angelica root, which "gave her some present ease." Elizabeth felt well enough to accompany her parents to afternoon church services, and seemed fine that evening. But in the middle of the night, things changed. Elizabeth woke her father, clutching her stomach and crying. Her pain had a very specific cause: "Father help me, help me, Goodwife Ayres is upon me she chokes me, she kneels on my belly, she will break my bowels."[33]

Even so, the Kellys thought the child's illness had a natural cause. They continued to use "what physical helps we could obtain" to cure their daughter, and more tellingly, they invited Goodwife Ayres, along with two other women, Goodwife Whaples and Rebecca Greensmith, to watch with her. When Elizabeth set eyes on Goodwife Ayres, she began to cry out again, saying, "Goodwife Ayres why do you torment me and prick me?" However, Goodwife Whaples did not take the girl's accusations seriously. She scolded Elizabeth, saying, "Child you must not speak against Goody Ayres, she comes in love to see you." Elizabeth presently fell asleep, and Goodwife Ayres said to the distraught parents, "She will be well again I hope," and went home.[34]

Except for the child's accusations, this sounds like a typical sickbed, with a typical group of women helping to tend the Kellys' ailing daughter. The familiarity with which Goodwife Ayres went in and out of the Kelly house, Ayres's comfort in helping herself to the Kellys' food, and the comment of Goodwife Whaples that Ayres had "come in love" to see Elizabeth suggest that she was an intimate of the family, a close neighbor who often shared sickbed duty and other chores with Goodwife Kelly.

However, while Bethia Kelly tried to downplay her daughter's fears at first, the seed of suspicion had been planted. Goodwife Kelly had noticed that Goodwife Ayres had spoken alone to her daughter, and she and her husband John quizzed Elizabeth about the content of that conversation: "The child told us both that when Goody Ayres was with her alone she asked me Betty why do you speak so much against me I will be even with you for it before you die, but if you will say no more of me I will give you a fine lace for your dressing." Bethia Kelly then went to Goody Ayres and asked her about the conversation: "Thinking she promised her something I asked her what it was. The said Ayres answered a lace for dressing." That night, Elizabeth Kelly died. Her last words were "Goodwife Ayres chokes me."[35]

When the child died, the Kellys performed two tests—one grounded in folklore, the other in law. First, they asked Goodwife Ayres to handle Elizabeth's body before witnesses, and when she did so, the body "purged a little from the mouth." In folk belief, a murdered corpse would bleed afresh if touched by its murderer. This test would seem to confirm their suspicions of Ayres. They also asked for an autopsy on their daughter's body. The autopsy revealed "6 particulars" that the presiding physicians found "preternatural." Even with this evidence in hand, the Kellys sat on their suspicions for a year, until another woman, Ann Cole, began to exhibit symptoms of demonic possession and bewitchment. It was at this point that the accusations began to leap from woman to woman, and to focus on the women who had attended Elizabeth Kelly at her sickbed.[36]

One of the first women Ann Cole accused was Rebecca Greensmith, one of the women who was called to Elizabeth Kelly's bedside. Indeed, when Rebecca Greensmith confessed to witchcraft, one of the women she named as a sister witch was none other than Goodwife Ayres. At this point, every one of Goodwife Ayres's actions became suspect, from the initial offer to share her spoonful of hot broth, to the fancy dress lace she had promised Elizabeth in her final illness. The Kellys revived their suspicions of Goodwife Ayres and joined in the accusations of Rebecca Greensmith as well. Bethia Kelly now named as agents of Satan the very women she once called upon to nurse her daughter back to health.

As the panic escalated, other women began to suspect those who had shared sickbed or childbed or birthing room duties with them. One name that came up over and over again was that of Katherine Harrison, "cunning woman," fortune teller, and sometime healer. Harrison may well have been an obvious suspect for any number of reasons: her dabbling in the occult for one thing, and her status as a property-holding widow for another. Gossip about Harrison had been common for some years, and when the Hartford witch-hunt began, the rumors resurfaced. The accusations came from women who had attended sickbeds with Harrison.[37]

Two or three years earlier, in 1659 or 1660, Harrison had attended the deathbed of a respected older woman, Mistress Robbins. Harrison insisted on intruding at the sickbed when she was not wanted. The invalid's husband warned her "2 or 3 times" not to come, and yet she continued to "thrust" herself "into the company." The Robbins family clearly resented the intrusion. The husband of the dying woman composed "a writing relating to prove witchcraft occasioning the death of his wife." As time went on, the fears of the Robbins family grew. When a daughter of the family fell ill, her first thought was that "I am afflicted by some evil."[38]

These rumors and suspicions did not stay within the Robbins family circle. Alice Wakely, who had been part of the sickbed gathering, added her voice to those who accused Harrison. She gave a deposition concerning the condition of Mistress Robbins's body, claiming that during Robbins's final sickness, her body became "so stiff so that she and Goodwife Miggat senior could not move either her arms or legs." Goodwife Miggat also joined the chorus of accusations against Harrison and gave a deposition during the panic in Hartford.[39]

The suspicions that began at a little girl's bedside in 1662 thus had consequences that expanded like ripples in a pond. First the women who had been directly involved in Elizabeth Kelly's care were accused; then other women who had behaved suspiciously at other sickbeds. The ripples also expanded beyond circles of women and into the larger community. Men as well as women found themselves involved in the witch trials: as witnesses, as clerical "experts," and as accused witches themselves.

Joseph Marsh testified in the trial of Goodwife Ayres, reiterating much of the testimony given by the Kellys concerning Elizabeth Kelly's illness. Like Bethia Kelly, he repeated the words that Elizabeth spoke concerning Goodwife Ayres—that it was Ayres who tormented her and caused her illness and pain. Marsh also claimed to have overheard the conversation between Elizabeth Kelly and Goodwife Ayres in which Ayres promised the child a dress lace in exchange for her silence. Given the lack of privacy in most early New England houses, it is not surprising that Marsh overheard these conversations—if he was visiting the house for any reason, he was likely within earshot of the child's bed. However, under normal circumstances, he probably would have ignored or forgotten what took place there. It was the excitement of a witchcraft case that caused him to take an interest in the women's work of tending the sick.[40]

Even more closely involved in the witchcraft cases were the ministers called in to pronounce upon the afflicted victims. When Ann Cole fell into the strange behavior that would trigger the Hartford panic, four ministers came to her bedside to diagnose and discuss her case. In odd cases like Cole's, ordinary medical expertise—often the province of women—was replaced by extraordinary learning and theological expertise, almost always the province of men. Whereas in an ordinary illness, Cole would have been surrounded by a group of female peers, her witchcraft-induced fits attracted four learned ministers, to observe and describe her "extremely violent bodily motions" and her bizarre "Dutch toned discourse." The ministers also made a point of writing to their colleague Increase Mather in Boston, to inform him of Satan's inroads in Connecticut. When they did so, the ripples from the Kelly case reached over a hundred miles away, to another town in another colony.[41]

Finally, there was Nathaniel Greensmith, husband of Rebecca Greensmith. He too was deeply involved in the trials, as one of the accused. He and his wife were accused by both Ann Cole and the Kellys. Both of the Greensmiths were subjected to the "swimming test," in which their hands and feet were tied and they were thrown into the Connecticut River to see if they would sink. When they floated to the surface, their survival was used as evidence against them. The Greensmiths were convicted of witchcraft and eventually hanged. Once again, suspicions and accusations that began as part of women's work and women's role had consequences that heavily involved men as well.[42]

Like many social structures in seventeenth-century New England, women's medical communities had a double edge. While they could serve supportive and empowering functions, the possibility of enmity and conflict was always lurking. In the case of Rebecca Greensmith, the women of her sickbed group literally hounded her and her husband to death. In the case of Goodwife Ayres, they hounded her away from her home, her family, and her community and into exile in New York. While the consequences were greatest for the accused, the events set in motion at Elizabeth Kelly's sickbed would eventually affect the entire community—and even touch people as far away as Boston. Witchcraft accusations are an admittedly extreme result of women's sickbed conflicts. However, they demonstrate that the forced intimacy of childbirths and sickbed gatherings bred fear and hatred as easily as support and affection. Just as the supportive bonds that formed among the Parkman women, the Maynards, and the Forbushes helped to tie the people of Westborough to each other, so the women's medical networks in Hartford in 1662 were the source of division in their community.[43]

WOMEN'S NETWORKS IN THE LARGER COMMUNITY

In early New England towns, family and informal social networks were closely related. Colonists saw family, kin, and neighborly relationships as guarantors of community stability and social order, and created social and legal institutions to enforce this ideal. Women's sickbed and childbirth gatherings are one more part of this picture. The authors who created this dominant image of the New England town focused on the role of business and religion in creating communities. While women certainly participated in both of these institutions, they were usually on the periphery. The medical network was one structure where women were at the center. Like business relationships and the church, medical networks reinforced existing kin ties and created new relationships.[44]

That the women's community was intimately involved in the affairs of towns as a whole is borne out by the fact that women's communities did not involve only women. Men had a strong role to play in the formation and maintenance of women's social and kin networks. Men surrounded and supported women's work of childbirth and healing, even though they were not part of the postpartum feasts or the adoption of kin.

Indeed, the very act of "calling the women together" was a male task. When a woman went into labor, it was her husband's duty to fetch the midwife and the neighbors. In the vignette that opens this chapter, Ebenezer Parkman twice roused himself early in the morning and traversed the neighborhood in the bitter cold of late December—the second time on foot. While several times he recorded assigning one of his older sons the task of driving the women home in the sleigh or wagon, for each of his wife's travails Ebenezer himself fetched her attendants. Samuel Sewall also recorded predawn journeys to fetch the midwife or take her home: "Went home with the Midwife about 2 o'clock. . . . Met with the Watch at Mr. Rocks Brew house, who bad us stand, enquired what we were. I told the Woman's occupation, so they bad God bless our labours, and let us pass."[45] Clearly, there were deep social expectations that husbands would provide the female attendants their wives needed.

Men sometimes had small gatherings of their own, usually to pray, when women came to the house to attend a sickbed or travail. Samuel Sewall called a minister as well as the midwife when his wife went into labor in 1702; while the midwife and women attended to Hannah Sewall's physical needs, Samuel and Mr. Willard together "called on God." At other times, men's prayer groups came to the actual bedside. When Sewall's mother-in-law was dying in 1695, she was surrounded by the usual group of female kin, including her daughter and granddaughter. Later, however, she asked that Samuel, her minister, and Dr. Oliver come to her chamber. Samuel and the minister prayed with her; the doctor prescribed a plaster to relieve the pain in her stomach. Close male associates participated in some of the same bedside rituals as female relatives, as when Ebenezer Parkman helped his mother-in-law undress his gravely ill wife, Molly, and put her to bed. Parkman sent the maidservant for Granny Forbush, then paced the room and prayed while his mother-in-law held her daughter's hand.[46]

Male household heads also served as intermediaries between female healers and learned physicians. Just as it was the husband's duty to call the midwife, so it was his duty to fetch the physician if necessary. In the scene above, Ebenezer Parkman sent for Mr. Barrett after Granny Forbush and Mrs. Whitcomb had dealt with the immediate crisis in Molly's health. Ebenezer wrote that he "said and did very little": He examined Molly, expressed his approval of what the midwives had done, and prescribed fennel and red wine for her fever. Afterward, he and Ebenezer prayed together. Significantly, Mr. Barrett did not work directly with the midwives and women but relayed his instructions through Ebenezer. He kept his practice and those of the midwives separate, using the patient's husband as an intermediary. He participated in the medical crisis but respected the boundaries of women's practice surrounding the sickbed.[47]

There was another way in which men served as go-betweens for physicians and female healers. Some doctors consulted with patients by letter, sending advice and sometimes medicines long distances.

John Winthrop Jr. conducted much of his practice in this way. The majority of letters to Winthrop that remain were written by men, even when it was a woman who requested the advice. Typical of Winthrop's correspondence is the following: "Sir," wrote William Leete in 1658, "you were pleased to furnish my wife with more cordiall powder by John Crane, for Graciana."[48] Similarly, John Pynchon wrote, "These lines are to request your advice and help in the behalf of my wife."[49] Men's greater literacy is an obvious explanation for these mediated requests. But there is probably also a cultural relationship between men's role in fetching physicians and midwives and their role in writing letters requesting medical advice. Women performed the intimate tasks of the birth chamber and sickroom, while men ensured that they could perform these tasks by dealing with the outside world.

The close relationship between the medical gatherings of men and women also meant that men's and women's gossip and social networks overlapped. Sometimes this intersection had immediate consequences for the sick person. Ebenezer Parkman heard from his wife's caregiver, Hepzibah Maynard, that a physician named Thomas Williams was visiting at the Maynards' house. Parkman duly asked Hepzibah Maynard to send Williams to see his wife.[50]

In other cases, the intersecting gossip networks had other effects. Nathaniel Smith was buttonholed by the suspected witch Rachel Fuller and asked for news, specifically news of the new physician in town, Dr. Reed. When Smith said he had no news, Fuller supplied some of her own—that she and her sister witches had abducted Dr. Reed and "led him a jaunt" with an enchanted bridle. This exchange later played an important role in Fuller's trial for witchcraft.[51]

The interaction between men and women in households where someone was sick or lying in and the movement of gossip from women's bedside to men's prayer circle meant that women's medical networks were tightly integrated into routes of communication. Such intersections of men's and women's community groups had important consequences for the function of women's medical networks.

THE FUNCTION OF WOMEN'S COMMUNITIES

Women's medical networks served special purposes for their members. The relationships that developed made it possible for women to take advantage of the social networks formed in birthing chambers and sick-rooms. Some women used the networks to resolve disputes to their own advantage; others passed information they gathered at sickbeds to their menfolk for further action. The narratives that follow provide case studies of the different ways medical networks functioned for women.

Loyalties within the women's community were complex. Women's responses to others in the network could be—and often were—influenced by other relationships. Women tried to solve their problems among themselves, but issues in the larger community intruded into the birth chamber and sickroom. Even so, these various loyalties did not stop some women from trying to manipulate the temporary solidarity of the birthing room to their own advantage. A set of two bastardy cases from Ipswich, Massachusetts, illustrates this point.

In 1686, Sara Savory and Sara Davis were pregnant out of wedlock. The putative fathers—Caleb Hopkinson in Savory's case, and Nathaniel Aylor in Davis's—denied their paternity. Both cases ended up before Magistrate Nathaniel Saltonstall, and Saltonstall required both men to pay child support despite their protests. The success in extracting support from the reluctant men came from the ways the women manipulated the women's community and the role of women at childbirth gatherings.[52]

In the case of Sara Savory, there does seem to be some doubt that Caleb Hopkinson was the father of her child. She had kept company with an Irish laborer the previous summer, and a neighbor had noted "uncivil carriages" between them. However, the laborer was penniless, and Hopkinson was well-off and could guarantee a steady stream of support for the child. Thus, when Sara Savory went into labor, her mother, Goodwife Savory, did not call a midwife. Midwives were bound to perform a formal "examination" of an unwed mother at the most painful point of her labor. Since it was a common belief that a woman could not lie under these circumstances, the Savorys did not want to run the risk of a midwife's presence.[53] Instead, Goodwife Savory conducted the birth and Sara's examination herself. As was customary, she also gathered a group of women at Sara's bedside, women who, unlike a midwife, were not quasi-official members of the court. Goody Savory and her daughter counted on the women in the birth chamber to support their story.[54]

The birth chamber was one of the few places where women could escape male authority. In a sense, childbirth customs were a form of sex role reversal. Women's traditions of birth and lying-in removed a woman from the day-to-day work of supporting her husband; instead, he had to cater to her needs. In a small way, this role reversal was a kind of resistance to the strictures that normally bounded women's lives. In the case of Sara Davis's and Sara Savory's illegitimate births in seventeenth-century New England, there was a special reason for using the women's community as a form of resistance. In New England in the 1680s, a transformation in attitudes toward fornication and out-of-wedlock births was underway. Men were beginning to resist taking responsibility for their sexual transgressions. The 1680s saw the origin of the sexual double standard that would reach full fruition in the mid-eighteenth century. When Caleb Hopkinson denied his paternity and threatened to leave Sara Savory destitute, she turned to the women's community to support her version of events.[55]

As soon as the women arrived at the Savory house, and well before Sarah reached "the height of her travail," Goodwife Savory asked her daughter gently to name the father of her child. "My dear child," she said, "search the trewth and wrong not thy soull or any innosent person." "Dear mother," Sara replied, "it is Goodman Hopkinson's child." Goodwife Savory turned to the assembled women and said, "You hear what she saith. You are all witnesses."[56] Sara had named Goodman Hopkinson in front of a group of women, all of whom could be relied upon to recount the scene as they had arranged it. The Savorys did not expect to be questioned by any of the women.

However, the women's community was not the only group involved here. The women at Davis's and Savory's travails had a variety of connections in the town, and they did not leave those loyalties at the birth chamber door. Men also heard about the conversations and gossip at the bedside and used that information for their own purposes. This intersection of men's and women's social networks was apparent even at the bedsides of the young women while they were in labor. When Goodwife Savory gently asked her daughter who the father of her baby was, her unorthodox "examination" did not go unchallenged.

One of the women in attendance, Goodwife Woostin, had been talking to Caleb Hopkinson and demanded that the Savorys conduct a more rigorous examination. "As much as you affirm it, he denies it," she said when Sara named Goodman Hopkinson. "He tould me he is as clean of the gilt of this thang as I am." "Hold your tongue,"

Goodwife Savory snapped at her. Goodwife Savory then tried to salvage her daughter's story. She had her daughter name Caleb Hopkinson again, saying, "You are all witnesses," to the assembled women. When Goodwife Woostin tried to speak again, Goodwife Savory put her hand over Goodwife Woostin's mouth to prevent her.[57]

There was a similar scene at Sara Davis's delivery when her mother tried to conduct a formal "examination" of Davis. In this instance, however, Davis's older, married sister came to her rescue, saying, "Let her alone now mother, she is in trouble enough now."[58] Goodwife Davis backed down. Elizabeth Woostin and the elder Goodwife Davis had their own reasons for doubting the "official" version of events. In Woostin's case, she had a relationship with Caleb Hopkinson that meant she trusted his word over that of the Savory women; Goodwife Davis surely had enough experience with her own daughter to know when to doubt her word. Although the peer pressure of the childbed gathering quashed their protests, the women's dissent illustrates how outside relationships and concerns entered the birthing room.

Despite the objections of Goodwives Woostin and Davis, the young women's strategies to obtain child support succeeded—at least at first. Although both Caleb Hopkinson and Nathaniel Aylor challenged their paramours' claims in court, Magistrate Saltonstall believed the women. He assigned legal fatherhood and child support to Hopkinson and Aylor. Most of the childbirth attendants supported Davis's and Savory's versions of events. The two young women were counting on that support, and on the whole, their assumptions were justified. While birthing room solidarity was not perfect, it was enough to get Davis and Savory what they wanted.

However, the case did not end with Saltonstall's assignment of paternity. The disputes over the fathers of Davis's and Savory's infants became grist for the gossip mill, and eventually became issues in an otherwise unrelated lawsuit. The way the cases were used in the new lawsuit illustrates two points: the growing doubt of women's word when it came to the fathers of their illegitimate babies, and the ways in which the events of the women-only birthing room remained the concern of the larger community.

This sequence of events began when Sara Davis started to enlist her own connections in the larger community to support her story. It seems that she and Major Nathaniel Saltonstall—the very magistrate who would hear her case—had a close relationship. Davis felt she could count on that relationship when she became pregnant, and bragged about it to whoever would listen. Two women, Dorothy Roberts and Marah Singletary, reported that Davis said on several occasions that Saltonstall was "more like a father to her than a magistrait or judg" and would thus hear her petition for child support favorably. Saltonstall's actions at the court session seemed to bear Davis's story out: he saw Davis privately in his house rather than in open court; he allowed her freedom of movement, while other women and men accused of fornication were under house arrest; and he spoke to her gently and kindly, while he publicly scolded Aylor and called him a "rascal."[59]

Saltonstall's behavior, and his decision to believe Davis and Savory over Aylor and Hopkinson, became the subject of much talk in Ipswich. Some were incensed that these respectable young men had been subjected to the shame and financial burden of supporting illegitimate children. Others found the Davis and Savory cases to provide more evidence that Saltonstall was a judge who played favorites. Foremost among those who resented Saltonstall's decisions was a man named Robert Swan. Swan had his own reasons for disliking Saltonstall, chief among them that he felt he had been overcharged on his taxes. Swan was also Nathaniel Aylor's father-in-law. When Saltonstall assigned paternity of Sara Davis's child to Aylor, and publicly shamed him to boot, it was the last straw for Swan. Swan began denouncing Saltonstall and the actions of the Ipswich court in general, claiming that he intended to get his sons elected as selectmen, for then he could pay lower taxes and not be forced to support bastards. As evidence for the general corruption of the Saltonstall court, Swan cited not just the case of his son-in-law and Sara Davis, but the allegations against Sara Savory as well. Clearly the story of the unorthodox "examination" of Sara Savory and her relationship with the Irishman had reached Swan's ears. When Saltonstall charged Swan with "defaming the acts of the court," Swan brought Goodwife Woostin and others who had been at the Savory birth to court to be witnesses in his defense, as well as those who had witnessed Sara Davis's travail and heard her boasts of favoritism.[60]

Sara Davis eventually heard the news of Swan's denunciations of Saltonstall's decisions, and Swan's implications that both Davis and Savory were lying about their babies' fathers. She promptly confronted Swan, saying, "I nevere did you any thing," and demanding to know why he was marshaling evidence against her. Swan denied that there was anything personal in it and claimed that he only wanted to discredit Saltonstall. Davis replied, "Do what you wish so that you lev me alone." In the end, Swan did present his witnesses but lost his case, and was forced to make an abject apology to Saltonstall.[61]

Davis's response to Swan's lawsuit most likely originated in her sincere desire to be left alone. But the tone of her confrontation with Swan also implied something else. She asked him why he was using her case to discredit Saltonstall, rather than merely contesting his tax rate. What, in other words, was this man doing questioning women's business, rather than keeping his dispute between men? Part of the answer is that nothing was ever completely women's business. The women's medical community was a subset of the larger public world, and events in one part of the community had repercussions in another. But Davis's main point demonstrates the expectations that women had of women's gatherings at travails. She and Sarah Savory took their problems to the women's community because it seemed to be the safest and most reliable constituency from which to challenge the male-dominated legal system. But as Swan's attitude made clear, in the 1680s, a woman's word in court was open to challenge, by disinterested as well as interested parties. When systems of protection for women within the formal public crumbled, women turned to their own single-sex networks to defend their interests.

Women did not use their medical networks only to defend themselves against male-dominated institutions. Men's and women's networks sometimes worked together to intervene in community disputes. Indeed, medical practice and medical networks were often at the center of the conflicts and factional squabbling that characterized New England towns. In some cases, like one that took place in Marblehead, Massachusetts, in 1662, women practitioners used the information they gathered at sickbeds and births to encourage more formal, male intervention in a dispute.

Marblehead had always been a contentious community, a scene of ethnic and economic discord. When a family squabble escalated to violence, leaders of the women's medical community decided that the situation demanded intervention. They asked their husbands to bring their concerns to the attention of the local court. This case demonstrates the interaction of women's medical networks, men's networks, and the courts in resolving community conflicts.[62]

Richard Rowland had never gotten along with his in-laws. Before his father-in-law, James Smith, died, they fought constantly. In the words of one witness, "What outrages there have ben betwixt James Smith, disceased the father, and Richard Rowland Sonn in law, it is allmost matter of impossibility to relate." Even after James Smith's death, Rowland and his mother-in-law, Mary Smith, kept up the dubious family tradition: "Ever since the fathers departure [the violence was] continued by the abovsaid Rowland against his Mother." The neighbors were well aware of Smith and Rowland's contentious and sometimes violent relationship, but they chose to tolerate it, at least for a time. However, in the fall of 1662 they had had enough: Rowland finally had gone too far in his assaults on his mother-in-law and had inflicted serious injury. Yet the case did not come to court immediately. It took the machinations of the women's medical community to bring Smith's injuries to the attention of the court.[63]

The local women had been aware of Rowland's assault on Smith for some time. Seven of them provided vivid descriptions of Smith's injuries after Rowland allegedly struck her with a fence rail. Smith's fifteen-year-old granddaughter Mary Eburne was one of the first on the scene. Eburne "found [Smith] lying on ground, leaneing on her Elbow, nobody being with her but her son Rowland, and when she came to her she Complayned that her backe was broke, and she saw a raile lying on ye ground, neer her feet so I cryed out yt Rowland had killed my Grandmother." Three other women soon arrived on the scene. Together with Eburne, they slipped an apron under Smith's back as a kind of makeshift stretcher and got Smith into the house.[64]

One of the most vivid descriptions of Smith's injuries came from Elizabeth Legge, one of the women who helped carry Smith out of the field where the assault occurred. After getting Smith into bed, Legge performed a detailed examination of Smith, with the help of the local midwife, Wiboro Gatchell. Legge declared that Rowland had given Smith "her death's wound," and described a "lash over ye arme." Smith's worst injury was to her back, where she had an enormous bruise, which was "something blacke [as if] ye seare cloth had beene upon it." The other women who gathered at Smith's bedside confirmed this description, emphasizing the seriousness of the injury and calling it a "death's wound."[65]

Elizabeth Legge and Wiboro Gatchell, between them, made sure that Smith's injuries did not remain the sole concern of the women's medical community. Legge and Gatchell were logical leaders of the women's community: Legge was the wife of the wealthiest man in Marblehead, John Legge Sr., whose estate was valued at 316 pounds. Gatchell, as the local midwife, had authority that stemmed from her medical expertise. It is no coincidence, therefore, that the first men to examine Mary Smith were Legge's and Gatchell's husbands. Legge and Gatchell had decided together that the case called for more formal intervention.[66]

Some time after the assault occurred, John Legge Sr. and John Gatchell came to Smith's bedside and performed a formal "examination" of Smith, similar to that performed by midwives when questioning an unwed mother. They put the question to her:

> The testimony of John Legg Senor, who testifieth and saith, that goeing to the bedside to goody Smith I asked her how she did, shee said shee was very weake, and further said that her sonn Rowland had given her her death's wound and that shee should carry it to her grave, and that shee should not [torn] from the bed until she was carried out.

> The testimony of John Gatchell, who testifieth and saith that goinge to the beadside to goody Smith I asked her how shee did she said I am very ill I feer he hath given me my death's stroke.[67]

The formulaic nature of the questions and responses suggests that Legge and Gatchell's visit to Smith was more than a neighborly obligation. They were collecting formal evidence about the assault. Women brought Rowland's violence and the extent of Mary Smith's injuries to the attention of their menfolk. The men then pursued the case on their own, and brought it before the formal authorities. In this manner, female networks interacted with men's networks to intervene in community disputes, and women healers took it upon themselves to bring women's problems to male authorities.

The early American women's communities surrounding sickbeds and childbirths served special purposes for their members. The relationships that developed around medical care were never entirely harmonious—indeed, there were numerous instances where members of a sickbed group turned on each other. However, the ties some women made at medical gatherings, under some circumstances, could create a base from which women could fight many battles. Even those who did not go as far as Sara Savory and Sara Davis could use the networks for emotional and material support. Such communities did not always consist of a set of loving friendships in an atmosphere of social harmony, but the society of female peers was crucial for both physical and social survival.

Women's healing networks never worked in isolation. Men gathered the women for childbirth, prayed for successful healing, and negotiated with learned physicians for advice, medicines, and support. Because of these connections, the women's community that surrounded medical practice was a gateway to the more formal structures of authority in early New England towns. Women used other women in their medical networks as witnesses in court cases and as investigators of disputes. Once a woman made her case in the women's community, she had a constituency that carried her through the formal procedures of the court. She could convince women who had close ties to powerful men to come to her aid, or she could draw on the women of the medical community as authoritative witnesses to advocate her interests. Whatever the disputed issue, the women's community was an important resource.

[4]

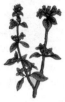

A Higher Calling

High-Ranking Women and the Uses of Healing

IN AUGUST 1659, AN EPIDEMIC struck New Haven Colony. Entire families fell ill at once. They were afflicted with excruciating headaches, high fevers, and delirium. Elizabeth Davenport, wife of the town's minister, John Davenport, was one of the few not affected. Carrying her satchel of herbs, she went from house to house, making soothing drinks, sitting at bedsides, and changing bed linens. She analyzed the urine of the sick and made herbal medicines that would bring the patients' humors back into balance. After several days, however, she began to fear that this illness was beyond her skill. She asked her husband to write to his learned friend John Winthrop Jr., requesting both advice and some of Winthrop's imported drugs.[1]

At first glance, Elizabeth Davenport's practice does not appear to be different from that of any other colonial housewife's. However, for community leaders, ordinary healing activities had additional meaning. In the previous chapter, we saw high-ranking women such as Elizabeth Legge and Wiboro Gatchell take responsibility to make sure the authorities intervened in the case of an assault victim. Other elite women saw their positions differently. Davenport used her medical skills to buttress her own standing and her husband's position as minister in New Haven. Ann Hutchinson used her medical and social leadership for a very different purpose: to challenge the religious and political status quo. Davenport's medical practice in New Haven Colony and Hutchinson's in Boston serve as contrasting case studies of the ways high-ranking women used their medical skills and their medical networks.

Elizabeth Davenport's husband John was a man of importance. He came from a gentry family and attended Merton College, Oxford, although he never received a degree. Before he emigrated to America, he spent several years as a private chaplain to an English noblewoman with Puritan leanings. After a brief stay in Amsterdam, he emigrated to Massachusetts in 1637. However, he arrived in the midst of religious and political turmoil and soon began looking for a site for a new settlement. He and his friend Theophilus Eaton entered into negotiations with the Quinnipiac Indians to buy a tract of land on Long Island Sound, and in April of 1638, they founded the New Haven Colony, where John Davenport became the first minister. He was more than just the spiritual leader, however; he "more than any other shaped [New Haven's] ecclesiastical and civil policies." In addition to performing his pastoral duties, he wrote numerous religious pamphlets and tracts. Historians know him for his theological conservatism and his fierce opposition to New Haven's union with Connecticut.[2]

Elizabeth Davenport herself left few direct traces in the historical record. Her own descendant, Benedict Davenport, wrote in 1851 that he had "never been able to ascertain either the maiden or Christian name of the wife of Mr. Davenport, or the date of their marriage."[3] While subsequent researchers have had better luck, she remains an elusive figure. Isabel Calder, who edited John Davenport's letters, discovered that Elizabeth's maiden name was Elizabeth Wooley and that she and John were married in England around the year 1619. Her name appears five times in the official records of New Haven. Once, she was a witness in a slander case; another entry records a small debt owed to her by Stephen Goodyear's estate. Other references register her place in the seating of the meetinghouse and mention (in passing) one of her illnesses.[4]

The best documentation of Elizabeth Davenport's life is in her husband's letters. John Davenport had a wide variety of correspondents, but one of the most important was John Winthrop Jr. John Davenport began writing to Winthrop in 1653 and wrote the last surviving letter in 1667. Winthrop was then governor of Connecticut. Many of Davenport's letters to Winthrop discuss health and medical matters. Indeed, the first letter he wrote to Winthrop in 1653 requested a consultation on his own health. Gradually, the content of the letters expanded to include many topics, including New Haven affairs, international politics, and religious doctrine.

Medicine remained a dominant theme in the letters, however. Twenty-two of the fifty-two letters John Davenport wrote to Winthrop discuss health matters. It is clear that many of the health-related questions in the letters came not from John but from Elizabeth. These requests were sometimes in a postscript: "My wife prayeth me to postescribe a word or tow concerning our maid servant . . . she had paine in her leggs." In other letters, it is apparent that it was Elizabeth's prompting that led John to write to Winthrop: "My wife desires a word or 2 of advice from you," he wrote in 1658. In 1660, during a time of widespread sickness, he stated, "I make bold, at my wife's request, to send my man with these lines."[5] There is also some suggestion that Elizabeth may have written to Winthrop herself. In a few instances, John makes reference to "enclosures" from his wife; unfortunately, none of these have survived.[6] From this evidence it seems that Elizabeth was as much Winthrop's correspondent as her husband was. It is easy to imagine her standing at John's shoulder as he wrote to Winthrop, describing symptoms and asking for Winthrop's advice.

Embedded in these requests is a rich description of Elizabeth Davenport's practice. She demonstrated a knowledge of household medicine that rivaled that of the Brigham family described in chapters 1 and 2. For instance, during one of her son's illnesses, in 1660, Elizabeth supervised all of his treatment. She prepared an herbal enema of fennel and mallows (among other ingredients) that would "open obstructions of the liver, spleen, and gall," according to herbals of the time. She prepared a poultice containing similar ingredients to relieve pain "in his short ribbes" and to reinforce the effects of the enema. Elizabeth also sat up and watched with her son, and proved an indulgent attendant. She catered to his whims, providing him with the "pap" of a baked apple when he begged for something to take the taste of medicine out of his mouth, despite her fears that the apple would undermine the effectiveness of the medicine. John Jr. "was exceedingly pleased wth the tast of it and did eate it with much delight." In addition to these commonplace abilities, Elizabeth Davenport had one skill that was unusual for seventeenth-century housewives. The letters contain a full description of Davenport's skill at interpreting urine for diagnostic purposes. During all of her son's illnesses Elizabeth provided full descriptions of the color and consistency of his urine, as well as mention of any sediment or other unusual qualities.[7]

Davenport used her medical skills at the bedsides of others as well, and formed her own medical network. This is where her situation begins to differ from that of other, more ordinary women. As women's medical networks acquired importance beyond their original function, they began to play important social roles within communities. Sickbed gatherings among women of Davenport's rank served as a reminder of the town's social structure in a manner similar to seat assignments in the meetinghouse.

Elizabeth Davenport attended sickbeds in New Haven with a consistent group of women. Mrs. Bache, Mrs. Goodyear, and Mrs. Jones turn up consistently at the same bedsides as Elizabeth Davenport. Not surprisingly, these women, like Davenport, were members of New Haven's most prominent families. Mrs. Jones was the daughter of Theophilus Eaton, New Haven's first governor, and the wife of William Jones, local magistrate and later deputy governor. Mrs. Goodyear was the widow of Stephen Goodyear, another deputy governor. Mary Bache's brother Samuel served on an important town committee with "ye governor & the magistrates & elders of Newhaven."[8] Most tellingly, Mrs. Jones, Mrs. Goodyear, and Elizabeth Davenport shared the first two pews in the New Haven meetinghouse, demonstrating that they were literally the first families of the town.[9]

These women nursed the sick of families equal in status to their own, following the lines of social, economic, and political power within the colony. Davenport brought medicines to attorney Joseph Alsop and to Nicholas Streete, her husband's assistant in the ministry. Perhaps most tellingly, she nursed Governor Francis Newman during his last illness in October 1660. She sat by his bedside, brought him beer from the ordinary, and made his medicines in her stillroom. Deathwatches like these were a visible reminder of who was who in New Haven—who had the privilege of seeing the governor into the next world, and who had to wait outside for the news of his death.[10]

Bonding with fellow elites was only one function of Elizabeth Davenport's healing work. She also visited the bedsides of those of lower rank, and in doing so, bolstered her husband's position. In 1659 she and her husband wrote to Winthrop concerning an outbreak of sickness in New Haven. Elizabeth had visited many of the town's households, dispensing medicines and advice, and sent the following description of the epidemic to Winthrop:

> Many among us are sorely visited and distressed, and some
> distracted, in the paroxisme of theyre disease, for a time,
> which taketh them in theyre heades with extreme paine, as
> sister Beamont, brother Myles and his son, his daughter also
> hath bene neare onto death, but I hope that, through the mer-
> cyes of God they are somewhat better. All John Thomas his
> house have bene downe, his wife is stil very weake, and him-
> selfe not strong, and all brother Doelitles house, excepting
> himselfe.[11]

The people mentioned in this letter were generally "middling sorts," judging from the location of their seats in the New Haven meeting-house. During epidemics, Elizabeth was busy in the community, going to any household who needed her. Indeed, much of the advice she requested from Winthrop concerned epidemic disease. In 1658 John wrote that Elizabeth needed to know "what is best to be done for those grypings and agues, and feavors." She made a similar request two years later, when there was "much sickness among us."[12]

Cotton Mather wrote in his medical treatise *The Angel of Bethesda* that healing was an essential part of the duties of "our Gentle-women": "The Wife of the Countrey-Minister should have some Skill and Will to help the Sick." Mather recommended that such women keep an herb garden for the preparation of medicines, and "have their Closetts furnished with several Harmless, and Useful . . . Remedies, for the Help of their poor Neighbours on Several Occasions."[13] With these words, Mather was merely confirming in print a tradition that women like Elizabeth Davenport had practiced for generations. In England, pious noblewomen like Lady Grace Mildmay and Lady Margaret Hoby were the main source of medical care for their tenants. Lady Hoby dressed wounds, performed minor surgery, and distributed herbal medicines. Lady Mildmay kept a medical notebook that contained advice for dealing with ailments ranging from sore eyes to epilepsy.[14]

Lady Mildmay ran a dispensary from her stillroom that catered to the poor and middling of her district, and gained a reputation for her skill. Like Elizabeth Davenport, she dealt with all ailments except those related to childbirth, perhaps because she felt that local midwives were adequate to those tasks. Unlike Elizabeth, she was able to dedicate large amounts of time and resources solely to her medical practice. Her stillroom was elaborate and so well stocked that its contents made it "resemble an apothecary's shop." More importantly, however, Mildmay viewed her medical practice as a religious duty peculiar to her rank. God charged the rich and noble to aid the poor and common. Grace Mildmay kept a devotional journal, even more elaborate than her recipe book, and dispensed religious exhortations along with her medicines.[15]

The tradition of the healing gentlewoman may have originated in England because only noblewomen would have had access to the education and resources necessary to practice medicine. The case of Lady Mildmay would seem to confirm this theory. Her education was more extensive than Davenport's and included the study of Greek and Latin texts. Grace Mildmay thus put her mental as well as her material resources to use when she opened her dispensary. Like their noble English counterparts, minister's wives in New England had more access to learned medical texts and networks of people who were willing to share their medical knowledge.[16]

Unfortunately, Elizabeth Davenport did not leave a journal like Lady Mildmay's. However, it seems likely that as a Puritan minister's wife, she was aware of the noble tradition of ministering to the poor and saw herself as filling that role among her husband's parishioners. The wives of other New England ministers cared for their husbands' flocks just as Elizabeth Davenport did. The wife of the Reverend John Cotton of Plymouth, Massachusetts, was active in caring for victims of a 1687 epidemic. She also sent "Advice and Directions" to those who requested them by mail, much as Winthrop did for Elizabeth Davenport.[17] The attentions of their ministers' wives reminded parishioners that their pastor was looking out for their physical and spiritual welfare. Davenport's medical practice served to support her husband's position, at a time when the ministry was as much a public office as a spiritual calling.[18]

This tradition combined with religious beliefs about sickness and healing reinforced the idea, held by both Davenport and Mildmay, that spiritual leadership required a concern for the physical. Tracts published in New England in the eighteenth century stressed that sickness was a particularly good time to turn a person's heart and mind to God. Like Cotton Mather's comments on the duties of the minister's wife, the sentiments the tracts expressed drew on older customs. They emphasized the spiritual side of sick visits, but they also urged readers to "be likewise suitably concerned for the bodies of your friends, when they are sick"; one reminded its readers that "sometimes persons are very sick and weak . . . and need much kind tendence and careful watching; in such cases, so far as our help is needed . . . we should readily give it."[19] Other tracts made a connection between visiting the sick and visiting the poor. Upon recovery from a serious illness, a good Christian should "immediately consecrate and set apart as a Thank-Offering to God, to be laid out in Acts of Charity to the Sick and the Poor."[20] The close association of spiritual with physical ailments, the special duties of the clergy to visit the sick, and the tradition of the English healing noblewoman all combined to make ministers' wives especially obligated to take their healing skills to the poor.

Thus, Elizabeth's satchel of herbs and other medicines reflected her prominent station as much as her medical skill. Caring for sick neighbors was a religious obligation that also reminded the community of her high status. This is one instance where the informal lines of power created at women's bedside gatherings supported the formal public power granted to men like ministers. As the compiler of Lady Mildmay's notebooks and journals noted, the fact that "the elite dispensed medical care . . . would reinforce the social structure—their succour to the needy helped legitimize their entitlement to rule."[21] Women healers like Ann Hutchinson used this power to promote their own agendas; more conventional women, like Elizabeth Davenport, used it to promote their husbands.

Davenport was able to use her husband's contacts to extend her medical network beyond the boundaries of New Haven. She could count John Winthrop Jr. as part of her network, in addition to Mrs. Bache, Mrs. Fairechild, and the other gentlewomen of the town. Winthrop had his own uses for the connection. Like Davenport, he could consolidate his own social status; also like Davenport, he had obligations to help those below him in rank. In Winthrop's case, he could serve both purposes by supporting Elizabeth Davenport's practice.

Winthrop was able to offer this support in part because the Davenports had great respect for Winthrop as both a man and a physician. The reasons for this respect began with Winthrop's European education. He did not have a doctorate of medicine, but he had attended medical lectures at the University of Amsterdam; in any case, Winthrop's education combined with his family background to raise him above most ordinary practitioners.[22]

More than formal education, however, Winthrop's self-presentation as an intellectual raised him above most artisan-physicians. He prided himself on being an all-around man of science and did his best to remain connected to the European scientific and intellectual community. His medical practice was deeply influenced both by the writings of Paracelsian physicians and by a personal correspondence with alchemical practitioners. The ingredients of Winthrop's medicines—saltpeter, mercury, sulfur, vitriol, and other chemicals common in Paracelsian and alchemical practice—reveal both these influences. In fact, a famous pseudonymous alchemical tract titled "Introitus Apertus, or Secrets Reveal'd" is believed by some scholars to be Winthrop's own work.[23]

Winthrop was also the first North American member of the Royal Society in London, a position that was a great honor. He wrote on a number of subjects in this role. He observed Jupiter with a homemade telescope and reported the possible existence of a fifth moon. He collected samples of New England plants and animals and sent to London preserved horseshoe crabs (unknown in Europe), hummingbird nests, and acorns. He conducted geological research with an eye toward the possibility of mining, and sent samples of New England beach sand along with an analysis of its composition.[24] Through Winthrop, Elizabeth Davenport was connected to the highest European medical and scientific circles. She thus had access to a pool of knowledge unavailable to other women and could take advantage of that knowledge when she tended her patients.

Both Davenports made it clear that they valued Winthrop's methods and drugs above those provided by other practitioners, female or male. Indeed, the Davenports manifested outright distrust of New Haven's resident physician, Nicholas Auger, and they often wrote to Winthrop to request a "better course . . . than Mr. Auger prescribed." The "course" the Davenports wanted most often was a dose of Winthrop's cure-all drug, rubila. Rubila was likely Winthrop's own invention. Its ingredients remain a matter of speculation, but Winthrop's biographer found the following list in the writings of Dr. Oliver Wendell Holmes: "It consisted chiefly of diaphoretic antimony and nitre in the proportion of 20:4; a little salt of tin may have been added, and there are hints of the presence of powdered 'unicorn's' horn. One can imagine yet other horrors."[25] The effect of this drug was that of a powerful emetic and purge—it worked both "upward and downward," as a seventeenth-century patient would have said. The Davenports had as much faith in rubila as Winthrop did himself, even though one of Elizabeth's herbal enemas may have been indistinguishable in effect. Only an educated man with overseas connections could prepare such medicines, and the rarity of its ingredients gave it an extra measure of desirability.

When epidemics struck, Elizabeth Davenport almost always took rubila to the victims, along with nursing care and her own homemade medicines. It seems that she was the prime source of rubila, which many in the town sought as a cure. In 1660, John wrote, "My wife also, having wholly spent your supply, is destitute of Rubila, which some have desired, but returned empty." Similarly, in 1658, John wrote on Elizabeth's behalf, to ask for more of "your powder" since "the supplye you left in her hand is spent." Being the main source of this desired medicine gave Elizabeth Davenport a certain amount of power over her neighbors, and demanded a certain amount of deference from those who needed drugs from her.[26]

Elizabeth Davenport needed Winthrop's prestige and his desirable medicines, but there is substantial evidence that he needed her just as much. Winthrop put Elizabeth in a considerable position of trust when she acted as an apothecary, especially since she explicitly acted in Winthrop's name. There are numerous references in the letters to this practice. In 1658, John thanked Winthrop for his advice and medicines "in distributing whereof my wife is but your hand, who neither receiveth, nor expecteth any recompence." In 1659 Elizabeth acknowledged the receipt of a "supply" of drugs "for the good of the people."[27] In his journal Winthrop recorded sending the Davenports large quantities of rubila and "powders" on several occasions. Elizabeth Davenport was, as her husband put it, Winthrop's "hand" in New Haven.[28]

The medicines did not just go in one direction, from Hartford to New Haven. Davenport also sent Winthrop medicinal plants for his own use. This aspect of their relationship began early in the correspondence. John mentioned in 1657 that he was sending along "the remaynder of the rootes [my wife] sent you before." When Winthrop himself was ill in 1658, Elizabeth sent "a few fresh raysons, and a litle licquorish, and your owne unicornes horne which she hath kept safe for you." John noted in this same letter that Elizabeth would be happy to send more medicines "but knoweth not what, til she heare further concerning you." The most specific reference to medicinal plants came in 1659, when John wrote the following postscript to a letter:

> The canded Comfrye-Rootes, which my wife sendeth to you are not so white as she desireth. The reason, she saith, is, because they were boyled with Barbados sugar, though clarified, yet they were canded with white sugar: but, she saith, they would have been whiter if they had been canded with loafe sugar. The tast nevertheles is good.[29]

Despite the description of the taste, this is a medicinal reference. A leading medicinal herbalist described comfrey root as being helpful in the cure of gout, moist ulcers, and gangrenes, as well as "ulcers of the lungs" and women's "immoderate courses" among other ailments. Winthrop's medical journal mentions the use of comfrey for several of John Jr.'s illnesses. Davenport grew and preserved the plants necessary to maintain Winthrop's practice.[30]

Davenport also supported Winthrop by providing him with crucial information. Her uroscopy skills enabled Winthrop to prescribe drugs appropriate to a patient's symptoms. Entries in his medical journal bear this out. For instance, during John Davenport Jr.'s illness in 1660, Winthrop noted the symptoms in his journal much as Elizabeth described them, and sent drugs chosen on the basis of those symptoms. The information Elizabeth Davenport sent meant that Winthrop could continue practicing medicine at a gentlemanly distance, without mucking about with urine flasks himself.[31]

All of this cooperation meant that Winthrop and Davenport worked together to care for the sick, effectively sharing patients. Winthrop recorded one detailed example of this process in his journal. In February of 1661, Davenport had been treating a young woman named Sarah Wilmott for "obstructed menses." While Winthrop sent chemical drugs and "salts" (meaning, perhaps, rubila), they were to be taken in combination with everyday household substances: Wilmott was to take a dose of salts "four mornings in beer" and four doses of saltpeter "in decoction with sage." Winthrop also specifically recommended that the first three doses of medicine were to be mixed with "the small brew of Mrs. Davenport," which may refer to plain beer, or to some mixture of beer and medicinal herbs that Davenport made.

A closer look at the instructions Winthrop sent demonstrates the mutual dependence of the two practitioners. Winthrop's instructions for dosages and combinations of drugs were quite complex. Wilmott had to begin her regimen of medicines by taking doses of "salts" for three days with Davenport's "small brew," then another medicine mixed with plain beer for four days, then saltpeter infused in a decoction of sage twice a day for four more days. Two months later, she was to repeat the saltpeter regimen for two days.[32] Such complicated instructions would seem to require some supervision to ensure that they were carried out properly. Elizabeth Davenport was the most qualified person to do this. Thus, even when Winthrop had taken over a case, Davenport's active involvement was necessary.

In this one case, the usual boundaries between male and female practice did not apply. "Obstructed menses" was a malady of the female reproductive system and usually would have been dealt with by a group of women. In this instance, Sarah Wilmott probably went to Elizabeth Davenport first, but Davenport felt, for whatever reason, that she needed outside advice. Since Winthrop was the person she usually consulted, she sent to him for instructions and medicines. Nor did Winthrop defer to female wisdom in this case—he promptly applied his own methods to Wilmott's complaint. Interestingly, he may have (wittingly or not) participated in an abortion, the ultimate women's business. However, in this particular case gender considerations were eclipsed by considerations of class. Elizabeth Davenport and John Winthrop could cooperate as equals in social status, and in this case erase the distinctions of gender that otherwise would have separated them.

John Winthrop's medical network was composed of a group of high-ranking women. Winthrop's relationships with these women were similar to the relationship he had with Elizabeth Davenport: they were equals in rank, but the women deferred to Winthrop as a man and an elite physician. Winthrop mentions in his medical journal women named Mrs. Newton and Anna Mason who seem to have had medical practices of their own. Both of these women were of social rank equal to or greater than Elizabeth Davenport. Anna Mason was married to Major John Mason, deputy governor under Winthrop.[33] Winthrop noted in his medical journal that she undertook to distribute his drugs in Norwich. In early May of 1657, Winthrop recorded sending sixteen doses of a medicine containing coral and anise; a month later he sent eight doses of "the same." At first, this appears to be for her personal use, but an entry directly underneath Mrs. Mason's suggests otherwise: "Beamont his family: I sent 32 [doses of medicine] to Mrs. Mason today . . . for them."[34] This entry, along with the large doses sent directly to Mrs. Mason, suggests that she was a practitioner rather than a patient.

Mrs. Newton was probably the wife of Roger Newton, minister in Milford, Connecticut, not far from New Haven.[35] She appears in Winthrop's journal as an active practitioner asking for help, much as Elizabeth Davenport did. Sarah Firman, an eighteen-year-old woman, had a sore eye, which "Mrs. Newton Useth to cure in 3 or 4 daies with oyle." The usual remedy was not working, and Mrs. Newton remembered that Sarah "had use formerly by a powder wc I sent hir to put in water."[36] Winthrop accordingly sent another dose.

So what benefit did Winthrop derive from his female medical network? The intangible benefits for him were similar to those accrued by Elizabeth Davenport in New Haven: support for his leadership in the colony. More specifically, the practice of medicine added to Winthrop's gentlemanly image. The indirect nature of Winthrop's practice was crucial to this image. Winthrop did the "head work," without any messy encounters with chamber pots or stained bed linen. A gentleman-physician did not dirty his hands, or use them at all. Nor could Winthrop ask a man of his own rank to do such work. Instead, women like Elizabeth Davenport, Anna Mason, and Mrs. Newton carried out Winthrop's instructions. In these examples, gender eclipses rank as the important hierarchy.

The prestige inherent in Winthrop's long-distance practice is evident in the great respect the Davenports showed for his skills. The deferential tone of the letters is so great it borders on the obsequious—despite John Davenport's own education and position as minister. This tone is especially strong in the passages in which John purports to quote his wife's own words, as when Elizabeth apologized for the color of the comfrey roots she was sending. More directly, Elizabeth demonstrated her respect by consistently consulting and deferring to Winthrop's judgment. As we have seen, during their son's two bouts with serious illness, the Davenports consulted Winthrop when Elizabeth was "fearful what to do." Elizabeth's need for advice permeates John's letters to Winthrop. During the epidemic of 1658, Elizabeth asked Winthrop for instructions because she "knoweth none whose judgement she can so rest in as yours."[37]

The Davenports further demonstrated their respect for Winthrop through extravagant thanks for his advice. After their son's recovery in 1666, for example, John wrote:

> Many hearty thancks being praemised, to God, and to you; to God as to the principal efficient, who stirred up your heart, and guided your minde to pitch upon such meanes as his blessing made effectual; and to yoursefe, as to a blessed Instrum[en]t in Gods hand, for our Recovery, my sons especially, from that weaknes, and those greate paines, wherewith he was lately and long afflicted, unto this measure of strength.

At another time, he asked Winthrop to "be pleased to accept our joynt thancks" for the medicines and advice Winthrop had sent. While John often expressed such joint gratitude, Elizabeth also declared her thanks on her own. In 1657, she asked her husband to send "a testimony of her readynes and desire to be any way serviceable to you." Such desires sometimes took a concrete form. Elizabeth sent gifts to Winthrop and his wife. In 1659, she sent "a small token of Marmalet of Quinces, which she hath made as good as she could, and hopes you boath and your daughter Mrs. Ann will find them to be comfortable for your stomachs and spirits." Such a gift was a "recompence [for] all your labor of love."[38] Even though Elizabeth may well have done most of the actual work, she gave credit to Winthrop for successful cures.

According to the historian Gordon Wood, "Ultimately, the rank of the 'better sort,' especially in colonial America, which lacked any legal titles for its aristocracy, had to rest on reputation, on opinion, on having one's claim to gentility accepted by the world."[39] Such reputations needed constant reinforcement. When a high-ranking woman gave a patient a medicine Winthrop had recommended, the recipients imbibed a reminder of Winthrop's rank along with a dose of physick. By forming medical networks with the high-ranking women of the surrounding towns, Winthrop made sure his claim to gentility was acknowledged not just by his Hartford neighbors, but throughout the Connecticut and New Haven colonies.

ANN HUTCHINSON

Not all high-ranking women used their status and medical skills to support entrenched social hierarchies. A few years before the Davenports settled in New Haven, Ann Hutchinson used women's medical networks as a base from which to foment explicit resistance to the established order. When Hutchinson began her spiritual campaign, she recruited her first followers from the women's community, specifically the groups of women who gathered to attend each other in childbirth. Like Elizabeth Davenport, Hutchinson used her connections in a women's medical community to create a social and political power base; unlike Davenport, Hutchinson used the women's community as a base in her attempt to subvert the social and political structure of Massachusetts Bay. Ironically, her main adversary in this quest was John Winthrop Sr., father of Elizabeth Davenport's friend and mentor.

Hutchinson is the most famous example of a female rebel in the colonial period, and her story is familiar to most students of New England history. She came to Massachusetts as a follower of the minister John Cotton, but soon developed her own version of Puritan theology that stressed the internal experience of God's grace over the outward appearance of righteousness and obedience to the authority of ministers. She acquired a large following in Boston. Eventually, the religious and political authorities of Massachusetts put her on trial for heresy and sedition, and she was banished from the colony and excommunicated from the church.

Hutchinson was a woman of unquestioned rank in Massachusetts Bay. She was the daughter of a minister and as a young woman had read widely in history and theology. She also learned extensive healing skills, either through her reading or from other women. She married a wealthy merchant, William Hutchinson, and moved to Massachusetts in 1634 with her large family. Hutchinson was then forty-five years old. Her age, her status as a matriarch, her skills as a healer, and her social rank all combined to make Hutchinson a natural leader among Boston's women.

Most accounts of Hutchinson's life mention that she was a healer or midwife, but leave it at that. Her contemporaries were well aware of her practice, however, and made much of it in their portrayals of Hutchinson. Her main adversary, Governor John Winthrop Sr., saw a connection between Hutchinson's medical role and her position as a religious agitator. When Hutchinson attended the stillbirth of a badly deformed child in 1638, Winthrop saw the event not as a commentary on the sins of the mother but as an indictment of the midwife and evidence of her spiritual "errors." Winthrop rather smugly noted that the child was born shortly before Hutchinson was banished from the colony. He also related that the parents and the other birth attendant were also justly punished. The parents were admonished from the pulpit, and the birth attendant was banished from the colony.[40]

Monstrous births were always taken as strong omens, but like other signs and wonders, they were open to interpretation. In many cases, a deformed child was read as an indictment of the parents' sin (as was the case when Hutchinson herself miscarried a defective fetus). However, the reading of signs and wonders was highly politicized, and interpretations were molded to suit the purposes of the interpreter. In this case, the "monster" reflected not primarily on its mother but on the midwife who delivered it. Hutchinson may have used the birth chamber to make converts, but in Winthrop's view she also got her just desserts there, in the form of a "monstrous" child.[41]

Some of Hutchinson's followers were also medical practitioners. Jane Hawkins, who attended the monstrous stillbirth along with Hutchinson, was a midwife and doctoress. Winthrop reported that Hawkins employed her medical skills to insinuate herself into the confidence of young women who came to her with fertility problems that she purported to solve. As with Hutchinson, Winthrop presented these aspects of her medical practice as evidence of her spiritual corruption. He used her fertility advice, as well as her attendance at the monstrous birth, as an excuse to have her banished. Her medicines to help women conceive contained ingredients such as mandrake root, which had long been associated with witchcraft, making Hawkins doubly suspicious.[42]

There are also more direct links between Hutchinson's medical practice and her religious rebellion. She used her status as a midwife and healer to recruit and retain converts to her own brand of Puritan theology. Both her erstwhile friends, such as John Cotton, and her sworn enemies, such as Winthrop, placed much emphasis on her medical skills in their accounts of the Antinomian crisis. John Cotton wrote in 1648, "At her first coming she was well respected and esteemed of me . . . chiefly for that I heard, she did much good in our Town, in woman's meetings at childbirth-Travells, wherein she was not onely skilfull and helpfull, but readily fell into good discourse with the women about their spiritual estates."[43] John Winthrop Sr. reported the same phenomenon, although he gave the situation a more sinister cast: "Being a woman very helpful in the times of child-birth, and other occasions of bodily infirmities and well furnished with the means for those purposes, she readily insinuated herself into the affections of many."[44] Both of these statements suggest the ways Hutchinson was able to use the atmosphere of the birthing room to create a social network that crossed lines of rank, and to use that network to attract women to her spiritual ideas. The intimate setting, combined with a birthing woman's natural fear for her own life, created an atmosphere that lent itself to spiritual discussions. Winthrop, among others, "marvelled that such opinions should spread so fast," but Hutchinson replied that "where ever shee came they must and they should spread."[45] A healer, with her reassuring skills, had power in the birthing room that went beyond the physical needs of her patient. This power, combined with her social status, made Hutchinson a charismatic leader. Hutchinson took advantage of this situation to spread her own subversive brand of theology.

At her trial, Hutchinson stressed that her ministry was to groups of women. She was an older woman instructing the younger, as justified by the Bible.[46] While she also ministered to a mixed group, these all-female gatherings were the beginnings and core of her following. Her original prayer groups overlapped considerably with her childbirth clients, and the nature of the groups themselves was similar. As single-sex groups, both bred intimacy: physical intimacy at the childbirth gatherings, spiritual intimacy at the prayer groups, and emotional intimacy at both. Hutchinson's leadership and authority were also similar in both settings. As a skilled healer, she took charge of difficult travails; as a charismatic preacher, she led her followers through spiritual difficulties and interpreted abstruse pieces of scripture.

Hutchinson seized on the two routes to leadership that were available to her as a woman: healing, and leading groups of women in prayer and Bible study. Combined with the deference due her rank, the forms of leadership fed back on each other and increased her reputation among the women of Boston. She was able to use her leadership role in the women's networks that grew out of travails and illness to recruit converts and establish spiritual authority.

Hutchinson's authority—and the threat she posed—went beyond religion and extended into secular matters as well. Her ministry occurred at a time when Massachusetts was engaged in a bitter debate over the nature of Puritan orthodoxy. The winner of that debate not only would guide the spiritual life of the colony but also would wield considerable political power. Hutchinson's followers were closely identified with one faction in this debate, a faction allied with John Winthrop's main political rival, Henry Vane. Furthermore, Hutchinson's ministry threatened the political power structure at a more fundamental level. Her challenge to religious doctrine comprised a threat to all authority—religious, governmental, and familial. Any challenge to the authority of the ministers, especially if initiated by a woman, was, in the eyes of Massachusetts leaders like Winthrop, a call to anarchy.[47]

As a member of this society, Hutchinson must have been aware of the provocative nature of her ideas. While there is no doubt that she felt her challenge was justified by God's word and her own religious conviction, she also knew that her dissent would require a base of supporters to make it viable. She thus began her ministry among those who would be most open to it—the women she tended in childbirth. She could use her authority as a healer and high-status woman to the best advantage among this population; she could also make converts in a setting where her male adversaries would remain unaware of her efforts for some time. The women's medical community provided a forum in which an ambitious woman could pursue her own ends. Hutchinson used the women's community to establish her own authority much as Elizabeth Davenport did, albeit with a very different agenda.[48]

Even after Hutchinson was defeated, the New England ministry acknowledged the power she had over her female followers. At her church trial John Cotton admitted Hutchinson's special appeal to women. He prepared a speech addressed specifically to the "sisters" of the congregation, "many of whom I fear have bine too much seduced . . . by her." He warned them of Hutchinson's theology but acknowledged the "good" Hutchinson may have done for them: "Let not the good you have receaved from her, make you to receave all for good that comes from her."[49] Even after Cotton disavowed Hutchinson and saw her banished, he felt the need to tread carefully when rebuking her female converts. Hutchinson's seductive powers had a lingering effect on women, and Cotton feared being too harsh with them. In an oblique way, this was an acknowledgment of the power of high-status women healers. The close association her enemies made between her medical practice and her religious ideas was an acknowledgment of the social and cultural power of the female healer and the gatherings that surrounded childbirth. Hutchinson used all of this cultural power to her own advantage.

Most high-ranking women healers were more like Elizabeth Davenport than Ann Hutchinson. They formed an invisible class that supported male healers like John Winthrop Jr. in their work as physicians and their rank as gentlemen. Despite what appear to have been long-term relationships, Anna Mason and Mrs. Newton merited only one entry each in Winthrop's journal. Elizabeth Davenport herself is only mentioned once—without her husband's letters, she too would have been lost to us. Indeed, it seems likely that even more women practiced medicine in cooperation with Winthrop, and that Davenport, Mason, and Newton were just three among many. That women's healing fades into the background should not be surprising. But the healing work of high-status women was a public function, similar to that performed when their husbands and brothers sat on the local courts and preached in the churches: it reinforced existing social hierarchies and provided a necessary service to the town.

Providing this service gave elite women a measure of authority and power. Some of this authority stemmed from their own skill as healers, but some was borrowed from their male peers and male cultural authority. Elizabeth Davenport acquired some respect in her own right, some from her husband's position, and some from her association with John Winthrop Jr. Asserting this authority required a delicate balance between self-promotion and deference to structured male power.

Ann Hutchinson chose to overthrow this balance. Instead of carefully making her way between asserting her own authority and invisibly supporting men of her own class, she chose to step aggressively into the public eye and claim power of her own. Her medical practice was one factor that enabled her to do so. Leadership in the sickroom and birth chamber reinforced her social leadership as a high-ranking woman. Both of these factors enabled Hutchinson to claim leadership in a areas normally off limits to women: religion and theology. While her mission ultimately failed, it remains as an example of the subversive potential of both high-ranking women healers and women's medical networks.

Other women healers also took their skills and their leadership into the formal public. Women practitioners were found not only at the bedsides of their families and in the homes of their neighbors but also in the witness box of the courtroom and in the commercial marketplace. These women chose to walk an even more delicate line between self-assertion and feminine meekness than did Elizabeth Davenport.

PART 2: *Authority*

[5]

Called to Court

Women Healers as Witnesses and Authorities

ON COURT DAY IN NEWBURY, Massachusetts, in the spring of 1670, Elinor Baily, a local midwife, waited to be called to testify. Ann Chase, an unmarried woman whose baby she had delivered, claimed to have been coerced into sex by a neighbor's servant. Baily had been skeptical of Chase's claims, especially as her labor stretched into its sixth day. If Chase were telling the truth, she thought, God would not prolong her travail. But Chase stuck to her story: John Allen had followed her out of the house, pinned her against a fence, and despite her pleas, gotten her with child. Even when Baily thought Chase was at the point of death, Chase insisted that this was the truth, even if she died for it. Finally, Baily was convinced. When she stood up before the judges, she would name John Allen as the father of Ann Chase's child. The judges knew Goodwife Baily could be relied on to recount the events of the birth chamber truthfully. Baily took some satisfaction in knowing that John Allen would face the consequences of his actions.[1]

Childbirth took place in a closed women's world. The court was a quintessentially male place. Under normal circumstances, these two worlds never met. But when an unmarried woman gave birth, or a woman was sexually assaulted, the two worlds came together. Women healers, especially midwives, shuttled between the the informal public of the birth chamber, the sickroom, and the kitchen, where the women's community went about its business, and the masculine formal public of the courtroom, with its official powers of government.

Early American courts have been compared to stage settings, where judges, plaintiffs, and defendants dramatized the values of the community. The dominant themes of these dramas were social hierarchy and masculinity. While many women participated in colonial court proceedings at some point in their lives, midwives and healers did so on a regular basis. Midwives in particular had specific, formal duties to perform. Through these duties, these women acquired authority and power that other women did not have.[2]

The privileged role of female healers stemmed from their unusual authority as witnesses. Court officials respected their opinions and relied heavily on their testimony in deciding cases. Unlike other women who appeared in court, midwives and healers had a considerable amount of autonomy in collecting and presenting evidence. The courts trusted their word. Much of this trust came from the court's respect for women's medical knowledge. Midwives, healers, and women who attended childbirths and sickbeds had a specialized knowledge of women's bodies, sexuality, and illnesses. In a sense, the women's medical community created a class of "expert witnesses" who could interpret female bodies in court.

Women healers used their special powers in a variety of ways. Some used their testimony to protect and defend other women; others used their court appearances to promote the cause of a particular community faction; and still others made sure that malefactors—both women and men—suffered the consequences of their actions. Midwives and healers were thus objects of both respect and fear within the women's community. A sympathetic midwife could protect a patient from the full wrath of the court, but she was just as likely to bring that wrath down, depending on her own judgment of the circumstances.

Despite this considerable power, healers' advocacy did have its limits, especially when compared to that of male physicians. Whereas women healers had more authority than other women, the scope of that authority was restricted to certain kinds of testimony in certain kinds of cases. Within these limits, however, women healers were able to make multiple uses of their authority, to champion their patients, their communities, and themselves.

THE SOCIAL RITUALS OF COURT DAY

The drama of court day did not serve only to settle disputes and punish criminals. As a social ritual, the actions of the court officials, witnesses, and litigants reaffirmed important values. Most writing on the role of the courts in enforcing the unspoken rules of colonial society focuses on the South, particularly Virginia. Despite the many cultural differences between the South and New England, these works make several points that also apply to New England courts. The colonial American courtroom was a place where "authority, law and custom mingled in ritual exchanges."[3]

The social function of court proceedings began with the physical space in which they took place. Courthouses and meetinghouses were designed to inspire awe and respect for order. Virginia courtrooms were decorated with portraits of English nobles and of the king himself. Seating arrangements, like those in churches, reflected social hierarchies: judges on a raised bench, wealthy men in front-row seats, servants and slaves banished to the porch.

The court did more than just impress the people with its own importance. Legal procedure and the social rituals that accompanied it affirmed the broader values of the society. Court decisions in Virginia reiterated the obligations of high-status people to low-status individuals, served as a community forum for shaming wrongdoers, and reminded servants and the poor of the deference they owed their betters. New England judges often prefaced their decisions with an affirmation of the value of social harmony and a peaceful, orderly society, as well as their obligation to enforce Christian discipline on those who disrupted this harmony.[4]

The social values of a court could have an important effect on its attitude toward women. The Christian basis of Puritan jurisprudence made New England courts more welcoming to women than the more secular courts of England and the American South during the seventeenth century: participating in the proceedings did not require special training or expertise; wives as well as husbands were encouraged to testify in cases that affected the family as a whole; and women crime victims were more likely to be believed.[5]

This is not to say, however, that New England courts were primarily women's territory or that they were bastions of sexual equality. Early New England court-day rituals, much like those in the South, dramatized formal, masculine power and authority. In one town in Maine, court day began with a procession of court officials from the town common to the meetinghouse, accompanied by the tolling of a bell and the beat of a drum. After a prayer and a court-day sermon, the procession re-formed and marched to the local tavern where the court proceedings actually took place. The public procession drew attention to the authority of the magistrates and judges; the sermon and prayer backed their secular authority with religion. Setting the court proceedings in a tavern added to the implicit enactment of masculinity, since taverns were sites of primarily male social life. When the tavern was set up for court—with the six justices solemnly arranged on a raised platform and the grand jurors seated below them—it embodied not just masculine social life but the intensely masculine nature of formal public power.[6]

Even when the court proceedings did not take place in taverns, the same aura of masculine prerogative surrounded them. In New Haven, depositions were taken in the front parlor of the governor's own house; formal court proceedings took place in the meetinghouse on the town green. Later in the town's history, the court moved to a specially built courthouse, whose design echoed the elaborate structures of Virginia.[7] Even though women were frequent participants in New England court proceedings—as petitioners, executors of wills, witnesses, and criminal defendants—the court itself remained a masculine space. As in the southern colonies, court-day rituals dramatized social order, political power, and by implication, masculinity. When a woman came to court to testify, she had to enter this alien place. Yet midwives and female healers had a surprising amount of respect, authority, and autonomy in this world.

Both male and female healers had the respect of the court. In the case of Hugh March, the ailing servant boy, a male physician, John Dole, described the boy's condition (the dispute between his mother and his mistress over his care is discussed in chapter 2). Hugh was "sick of a fever, and also a tumor or swelling in his knee."[8] In another court case, the physician Philip Reade was called to examine the injuries of two murder victims and concluded that the wounds had been inflicted "as i conseve . . . with the pole of an Ax."[9] The court depended on doctors' testimony for neutral descriptions of injuries and illnesses and placed a great amount of trust in their honesty and expertise. As we will see, the same weight was given to the testimony of midwives and other women healers, albeit in different kinds of cases.

Courts and other authorities demonstrated their respect for healers, both male and female, in their official acts. Some towns provided incentives for reliable practitioners to settle in their communities. In

1651, the town fathers of New Haven offered to build a house for Dr. Chaise if he agreed to live and practice in their town. The same town council provided the midwife Widow Bradley with a house and "farm lot" rent-free in 1655, since she had proved "verey helpfull, specially to ye farmes, and doth not refuse when called to it." Four years earlier, the town had paid to build a fence for the midwife Hannah Potter and to repair damage to her house.[10]

Other women healers received special treatment when they found themselves in trouble with the law. When Rebeckah Potter committed fornication, her paramour was sentenced to be whipped; Potter, however, was spared this punishment. "Considering her worke as a nurse," the court declared that "she only pay two pound ten shillings fine to the treasury, & stand by John Tharpe when the sentence is inflicted on him."[11]

Healers had a special position in the court, but in some medical matters, laypeople were asked to perform quasi-medical duties. Women's roles in these medico-legal proceedings diverged from men's roles in important ways, and the ways in which they differed outlines the basis for women healers' legal authority. All women were thought to have special knowledge of women's bodies that men—even learned men—did not have.

There were two kinds of quasi-medical juries. Juries of inquest, created to investigate suspicious deaths, were composed of laymen. Courts appointed groups of laywomen to act as "searchers" to examine women's bodies, for witch marks, for signs of pregnancy, and for evidence of injuries inflicted during the course of a crime.

While the female searchers and male jurors of inquest resembled each other in some respects, there were subtle differences in their duties. Whereas male jurors of inquest sometimes physically examined cadavers, they were most concerned with the circumstances of the death: was this an accident, a suicide, or a murder? Therefore, inquest juries spent most of their time interviewing witnesses and looking at other kinds of evidence. Their official verdicts often mention physical injuries only peripherally: "Haveing seene and considered ye place of ye river where ye sayde childe fell in, and spoken with such as could give any evidence in the case, doe . . . give it as our verdict that ye sayde childe . . . probably fell out of a canoe where he was playing alone."[12] When more explicit medical expertise was called for, the court called on a physician or surgeon.

Women's matron's juries or searchers were created specifically to give opinions about women's anatomy and the physical condition of female victims or defendants. Unlike male jurors of inquest, laywomen were assumed to be familiar enough with women's bodies to render important legal judgments. The most dramatic use of searchers was in witchcraft trials. In these cases, courts usually appointed a "jury of matrons" to examine the accused for witch's teats and marks. The first record of a court appointing a matrons' jury in England was in 1579, when the male jury specifically requested such a search; however, it seems likely that the matrons' jury was a custom with even older roots.[13] In America, courts appointed groups of women in many witchcraft cases, including the Salem trials.

Even when male physicians were available to the court, groups of women performed the searches.[14] Male court officials mistrusted their own ability to judge what was a normal part of a woman's body and what was a supernatural growth. When Richard Ormsby, the constable of Salisbury, Massachusetts, whipped the suspected witch Eunice Cole, he noticed "under one of her breasts . . . a blue thing like unto a teat hanging downward about three quarters of an inch long." Naturally, seeing such a thing raised Ormsby's suspicions. Yet his first action was not to use his own testimony to indict Cole for witchcraft, but to ask "the court to send some women to look of it."[15]

The authority that laywomen enjoyed in witchcraft cases extended to other types of cases. Elizabeth Rinke, for instance, was called to testify in a 1656 Boston divorce case. At issue was whether the wife in the case was still capable of bearing children. Her husband claimed that "the corse of nautr in his wiff hath bin stopped for severall months." Rinke testified that the woman was still fertile: "The deponant hath observed her linen soe that I can testyfie the contrary and that she hath had the due course of natur upon her."[16]

THE LEGAL AUTHORITY OF FEMALE HEALERS

Other cases required other kinds of expertise. The most common and well-known legal duty of midwives was to question unwed mothers about the fathers of their children. Although this practice had ancient origins, it was formalized in the earliest written law of the New England colonies. The statutes of Connecticut, New Haven, and Massachusetts Bay had similar wording: a woman pregnant with "a child which if born alive may be a bastard" must be "put upon the discovery of the truth respecting the . . . accusation in the time of her travail."[17] In the early years of the New Haven Colony, the lawmakers were most explicit in supporting this practice with the idea that women would not and could not lie under these circumstances. While such trust in women's word would fade over time, this practice remained current through the early nineteenth century.[18] Indeed, the most common reason for midwives to appear in court was to testify to the identity of a child's father. If the midwife could not come for some reason, "somm sober woman or women, that was at her travell" could substitute.[19]

Midwives served as experts in other sexual matters as well, both in and out of court. The Gloucester, Massachusetts, midwife Grace Duch was called to interview a young maidservant who accused her master of sexual assault. When Duch arrived, Mary Somes was "crying in the Roome wishing herself dead." After some time, Duch extracted the following story from her, with the help of Somes's mistress, Goodwife Jackson: early that morning, Somes had been lying in bed, feeling poorly. Her master came into the chamber and "took his prevy members and put it into her hand and seed that [w]ould mack her well." This was not the first but the fourth time such an incident had occurred. Somes was only able to escape her master's attentions by biting his nose.[20]

The court records do not state why Grace Duch was the woman called to interview Mary Somes. Perhaps Goodwife Jackson merely thought that a woman trusted in the birth chamber could also be trusted to calm a hysterical young woman. But it is likely that Duch's authoritative role in court proceedings played a part in the Jacksons' choice of witness. Duch often appeared in court to testify to the examinations she had made of unwed mothers. This fact may have helped Duch get the story from Somes, adding a hint of intimidation to the questioning. Perhaps this is the role that Goodwife Jackson had in mind when she sent for Duch, hoping that Grace Duch could get the truth about her husband's behavior with their servant, just as Duch got the truth about the fathers of illegitimate children. The aura of legal authority hovered around the midwife even outside court, so that neighbors sought her out to witness events and take depositions. Whatever the case, Grace Duch was the woman who told Mary

Somes's story before the court. It was the midwife—not the victim, not her mistress—who testified about the incident.

Grace Duch's quasi-official role even outside the courtroom suggests another important point. The respect, authority, and autonomy women healers had in the courts gave them access to community power that few other women had. They had the ear of the court and a reasonable expectation that their testimony would be believed and acted on. Midwives and healers were thus able to use the courts to their own advantage. Given that they were called upon to "officially witness" many disputes, they had considerable leeway to act as advocates. Healers could choose which side of a community dispute they would present in court. When they did so, they had considerable influence in determining the outcome of the case.

A 1657 witchcraft case from Gloucester, Massachusetts, is a good example. Witchcraft accusations were often the culmination of months or even years of factional infighting within a community. After a period of escalating tensions, a member of one faction would accuse a member of the other side of witchcraft. The case in Gloucester was no exception in that regard, although in a reversal of the typical pattern, a group of women leveled the main accusation against a man. William Browne was accused by Margaret Prince and her women's network, which included several midwives.[21]

The dispute that engendered the ultimate confrontation between Margaret Prince and William Browne had a history that traced back to the founding of Gloucester. The first minister of Gloucester, Richard Blynman, had left the community for Connecticut in 1651 under a cloud of financial scandal and religious antipathy. Since then, Gloucester had had no minister. Instead, it had a series of "teaching elders." William Perkins had been the first, but he left the post after five contentious years; Thomas Millet replaced him, but his preaching had not appealed to the congregation any more than that of Blynman or Perkins. Millet had to sue the town to collect his salary and fend off complaints from another church member that he had acquired his post through illegitimate means. These religious disputes dispersed into the community as a whole. Everyone had an opinion, and everyone took a side.[22]

The court record in the Browne witchcraft case begins with a description of Browne's behavior leading up to his confrontation with Prince. Clearly, Browne had strong opinions about the town's ministerial situation and was not afraid to express them to whoever would listen. In Margaret Prince's presence, Browne spoke "disgracefully" against Blynman, Perkins, and Millet, saying "Mr. Blinman was naught, and Perkins was stark naught, and Millet was worse than Perkins."[23] It becomes clear through the rest of the testimony that the pregnant Margaret Prince was on the opposite side of this dispute. Tellingly, Browne asked Prince if the "parson had not been here to feel [her] belly whether [she] were with child of a boy or a girle," an accusation that managed to imply that Thomas Millet and Margaret Prince were dabbling in both sexual impropriety and the supernatural. Even more tellingly, Browne tried to coerce Prince into removing her name from some piece of paper she had signed—perhaps a petition concerning the latest development in the ministerial saga. Finally, it should be noted that Mrs. Millet, the wife of the parson, had attended Margaret Prince in childbed and thus was a member of Prince's medical network.

Browne accused Prince of being "divided against hir husband," noting that her husband had not signed the disputed "paper." As the argument escalated, he threatened to send her to the devil "for a new year's gift" and to see her "beg her bread" before she died.[24] Immediately after Browne cursed her, Goodwife Prince fell into travail and began to bleed. After six days of fruitless labor, the assembled women gave her up for dead. While Goodwife Prince eventually recovered, her infant was stillborn. The women at once accused Browne of murdering the Prince infant by witchcraft.

Testimony in Browne's defense centered around two points: first, that Goodwife Prince had indeed rebelled against her husband, and second, that Goodwife Prince had brought on her premature labor by performing physical work that was too strenuous for a pregnant woman. Thus, medically, the midwives could take either side. They could testify that this was an ordinary stillbirth, brought on by Prince's irresponsible behavior, or they could declare that this was an "unnatural" event brought on by Browne's diabolical powers. The choice they made in their testimony was a political one, since the outcome of this case would be one more event in the ongoing factional dispute in Gloucester.

The midwives came down on the side of Margaret Prince, and by extension, in support of Mr. Blynman, Mr. Perkins, and Mr. Millet. The birth attendants said over and over again that there was no "natural" reason for Goodwife Prince's trouble and the death of her infant.

Their testimony had two purposes: to convince the court that the supernatural was involved in Goodwife Prince's condition, and to contradict evidence that Goodwife Prince had brought the early labor on herself. The evidence for the latter contention was particularly strong: Browne produced a woman who had seen Goodwife Prince carrying heavy buckets of clay to seal cracks in the walls of her house. Worse yet, the witness had seen her carrying the pails on her head. If a pregnant woman raised her arms above her head, it was thought to tangle the umbilical cord and possibly kill the fetus. Thus, the midwives were emphatic in their testimony that Margaret Prince's labor was far from normal—that it was, in fact, supernaturally complicated. For the first four days of the ordeal, Goodwife Prince's travail was "contrary to other woemen in that condition." Isabel Babson, one of three midwives present at the birth, was "troubled . . . to see the woeman so full of pain." Most disturbing was the bleeding that accompanied the contractions, a condition that was "not usual."[25]

Goodwife Babson and the other midwives, Grace Duch and Elinor Baily, took special care to point out that the condition of the fetus was completely outside their experience. Goodwife Duch and Goodwife Baily both testified that the fetus appeared to be "whith out spott or hurte," except that it "had no bloud in it."[26] Isabel Babson confirmed this account. She further said that the baby died "without any hands of woeman." "All of us did what they coulde to preserve the life of mother and childe," she said, and she could see no reason why the baby should have died beside "william Browne shakinge his hand against the wife of Thomas Prince."[27] All three women added that when William Browne entered the Princes' house, the baby's corpse bled from the nostrils, a sign that its murderer was in the room. This sign had further significance given that the women believed that the baby's body had no blood in it at birth.

The midwives crafted their advocacy primarily to support Prince's side in the ministerial controversy. However, they also did as much as they could for Margaret Prince personally. During the confrontation, Browne had accused Prince of being "one of Goodwife Jackson's imps," linking her with a woman who had a strong reputation for witchcraft herself. He had also stated that she was a shrewish wife who openly opposed her husband in questions of religion.

The birth attendants did their best to defend Prince's reputation from harm. They took aim first at the implication that Prince was a disloyal wife. Isabel Babson said that Goodwife Prince's greatest fear was that Browne's words "should breed some disquietness" between herself and her husband. This suggestion "did more trouble her then all the rest."[28] A neighbor woman who saw Goodwife Prince shortly after Browne cursed her noted that "all men should take warninge how they did lett any men to abuse their wives."[29] To refute Browne's claim that Prince was a follower of reputed witch Goodwife Jackson, the birth attendants stressed their personal support for Prince and presented evidence of her Christian piety. They described how they had prayed together while they tried in concert to save both the child and the mother.[30]

The women of the neighborhood supported and cared for Goodwife Prince and thought she was a virtuous wife and a responsible mother. By so portraying her, the midwives and other women protected Margaret Prince's personal reputation from harm, and by extension lent credibility to their faction's position in the dispute over the leadership of Gloucester's church. In the end, however, the court chose not to award a clear victory to either side. Browne was never formally tried for witchcraft but did spend a week in prison, presumably as a warning against making more rash speeches in the future.[31]

In the Prince–Browne case, the midwives tried to bring the point of view of the women's community into the courtroom. In other cases, healers brought the values of the court into the sickroom. The authority midwives and healers enjoyed in the courtroom carried with it a responsibility. Midwives not only represented women's interests in court but also represented the force of the law among women.

Most often, the legal duties they performed were benign. Healers and nurses were trusted witnesses when heirs challenged a deathbed will, for instance. George Carr was so weakened by his final illness that he was unable to make a written record of his wishes. All he could manage was an oral request that his "children . . . agree amongst them selves."[32] Elinor Baily testified to these words and further said that Carr was not mentally capable of making a more elaborate will. Similarly, the New Haven midwife Hannah Beecher attended the deathbed of John Bishop and made a mental note of his desire to leave his meager property to Mr. Hooke and Richard Spery.[33] In cases such as these, women healers represented the property concerns of the court even as they comforted the dying.

In rape cases, the word of a jury of matrons could provide crucial evidence to support a woman's accusation. In Boston in 1673, twelve-year-old Sarah Lambert was raped by Peter Croy. In order to obtain a conviction, the court needed two witnesses to the crime—the victim and one other. Sarah had been alone, tracking down her master's cows in an isolated meadow, when the attack occurred. There was no other eyewitness, but there was the testimony of the midwife Elizabeth Weeden, forewoman of the matron's jury sent to examine Sarah's injuries. The jury "did finde that she has been abused by him." The court was satisfied with this conclusion and declared "it all amount unto two Legall evidence, then wee finde peter Croy guilty."[34] Juries of women could also lend weight to their testimony by expressing their moral outrage over a crime. A ten-year-old servant girl accused one of her fellow servants of rape in 1678. The women appointed to examine her, Grace Healy, Mary Bacon, Esther Cheaver, and Elizabeth Hicks, reported, "We do find her body hath been greatly abused by some wicked person. . . . And . . . wee find her body much rent and soare." To this damning evidence, they added in a marginal note that the victim was "as greatly wronged as is imaginable."[35] In these cases, when a midwife combined her legal authority with her medical expertise, it worked to the advantage of the female victim, and when the midwives were convinced of the perpetrator's guilt, they did all they could to ensure his conviction.

Yet the healers' role as officers of the court was not always so benevolent. If the jury women did not believe that a rape had taken place, they abandoned their sympathy for the victim. In a case from Woburn, Massachusetts, the midwives called to examine Elizabeth Pierce (or Pearce) pressed her hard on the details of her story: "We asked Elizabeth Pearce whether his breaches was down she said to us his breaches was not down wee asked her also why she did not cry out she said she durst not for fear he would knock her head and we asked her if he had any thing in his hand and she said he had nothing." They extended their skepticism to their conclusions about Elizabeth Pierce's physical injuries. They were so slight, they said that "we cannot arrest the young man thereby," since the marks "might be the scratch of a pine [pin] for ought we know."[36]

As we saw earlier, midwives could be equally relentless in their questioning of unmarried women about the fathers of their babies. Like Elinor Baily in the opening vignette, midwives did not scruple at telling them that their labors were prolonged by lies. Adultery cases in particular demonstrate that midwives did not always choose to protect other women. Grace Duch supported Mary Somes in the dispute with her master and testified on behalf of Margaret Prince. Some years earlier, however, she had been the main witness supporting the indictment of one Goodwife Glover for adultery.[37] In a Marblehead, Massachusetts, case from 1682, Ruth Williams confessed to adultery with Peter Goite during her travail, but later recanted and claimed that the child was her husband's. The midwife, Wiboro Gatchell, and two birth attendants, Rebecca Sweet and Elizabeth Smith, testified that the child was Goite's. Sweet and Smith further testified that they "hath seen the said Goite goe into the Roome to sd Ruth at 12 or on o'clock at night, but did not see him when he went forth againe."[38] In this case, the women supported the folk and legal doctrine that a woman's word during travail was more reliable than at other times— the doctrine that formed the basis for much of their legal authority.

Such authority did not always go unchallenged. Given the potentially dire consequences of a healer's testimony, those accused sometimes tried to discredit midwives and other women who testified against them. Such challenges illustrate two points: the fear that a healers' opinions could engender, and the independence of the women's community in making certain kinds of medical judgments. Courts rarely interfered with such challenges, and when a woman felt threatened by a decision of a matrons' jury, it was up to her to challenge it on her own.

In a notorious witchcraft case from New Haven, Mary Staplies challenged the searchers' opinion to save her own skin. Rumors of witchcraft had followed Staplies for months. When another woman, Goodwife Knapp, was convicted of witchcraft, Knapp named Staplies as one of her fellow witches. Staplies then attempted to discredit the evidence that had convicted Goodwife Knapp, in the hope that she might be able to clear her own name of suspicion and save herself from Knapp's fate.

When Goodwife Knapp was hanged, Mary Staplies attended along with a great crowd of her New Haven neighbors. After the body was cut down, Staplies demanded to see the witch's teat that had played a crucial role in Goodwife Knapp's conviction. She and several members of the matrons' jury gathered at Goodwife Knapp's grave, where Staplies examined the body and found the supposed witch mark. She called to Goodwife Lockwood, who had been on the panel, and said, "These were no witches teates, but such as she herselfe had, and other women might have the same." Staplies seemed to imply that Good-wife Lockwood had committed perjury, by saying to Lockwood that "she had bine upon her oath when she found the teates." Other women from the jury came to look. Staplies pulled at the alleged teat and claimed that all women had such features, that she herself had one, and that so would Goodwife Lockwood, "if you search your-selfe."[39]

At this point, the assembled jury women began to fight back. Good-wife Lockwood declared that if she had such a growth on her own body, then she deserved to be hanged. Another searcher, Goodwife Odell, examined the mark and said that "no honest woman had such." Mary Staplies hesitated, still fingering the mark. Emboldened, the as-sembled women began "rebuking her and said they were witches teates."[40] At some point, the local midwife pointed out more specifi-cally which marks were unnatural. Staplies backed down and ap-peared to accept that the marks were indeed witch marks. While she was heard to say, along with Odell, that "no honest woman had such," it is not clear whether she was truly convinced, or whether the consid-erable pressure brought to bear by the midwife and other women finally intimidated her into withdrawing her claim.[41] It seems that Staplies fi-nally decided that to pursue her claim further would be counter-productive—that the challenge to the legal and social authority of the jury would only bring other legal consequences down on her head.

The way in which the dispute was handled is indicative of the au-tonomy of women healers in court cases. Staplies challenged the searchers' expertise directly, by confronting them at Goodwife Knapp's graveside with the disputed evidence, rather than challeng-ing them in court. The women of the panel responded just as directly, not referring to the authority of the magistrates but depending on their own expertise in female anatomy to convince Goodwife Staplies of Goodwife Knapp's guilt.

Mary Staplies and the jury of matrons did not bring their dispute into court because it was a dispute among women, concerning women's business. Such disputes did not normally end up in court-rooms but were informally resolved. Marginal groups, such as land-less men and servants, often used extralegal dispute-resolution mech-anisms. These groups preferred their own methods to those of the courts, which were controlled by the wealthy and powerful. The jury women here were following a procedure that women must have turned to often. In this case, women were able to use the strategy of the marginal to underline their autonomy.[42]

The informality and independence of the dispute did not mean the proceedings were not public. Indeed, Goodwife Staplies deliberately chose to make her attack on the jury in a place where the entire community was likely to see. If she was vindicated, she wanted to make sure that everyone knew about it. In addition, this public argument served another purpose. Just as court proceedings could be ritual enactments of social hierarchy or masculinity, the Staplies dispute was a ritual enactment of the authority of women's medical expertise.

Finally, this incident vividly illustrates the healers' role as enforcers of community norms. By helping to hang witches, convict adulteresses, and ensure the orderly passage of property, female healers took on some of the same duties of social control as the magistrates and judges themselves. Women healers who were not midwives also took their duties to enforce community norms quite seriously. They saw their duty as extending beyond sexual matters and witchcraft into other kinds of cases.

The widow Greenslet worked in Salem, Massachusetts, as a nurse. In 1680 she took on the job of nursing Isabel Pudeator, a notorious alcoholic. Widow Greenslet did her best to keep her charge from drinking and being a public nuisance, even though "she would have itt [rum] if itt was to be had for there backs could not be turnd, but she would out of doors & carry any thing wth her to pawne for Rum." When Goodwife Pudeator died, Widow Greenslet added her testimony to those who suggested that Goodman Pudeator had poisoned his wife by encouraging her to drink porringer after porringer of brandy. Greenslet's vocation carried with it the duty of social enforcement.[43]

At times the duty to act as an enforcer of values outweighed even medical obligations. The doctoress Ann Edmonds of Lynn, Massachusetts, turned patients from her door on two occasions when she judged them undeserving, despite the possible loss of income. In one case, she turned William Perkins away when he arrived so drunk he could not sit his horse. In this example, she behaved as Widow Greenslet did, although Widow Greenslet did not go so far as to condemn drunkenness by refusing to care for the drunkard.[44]

The second time Goodwife Edmonds rejected a patient was more complicated. In 1665, a young man arrived at the ordinary in Lynn, fresh off the ship from England. He complained that his body ached and that he was short of breath. He was flushed along the cheeks with fever and chalky around his mouth. Clearly, he was very sick. The young woman who served him beer, Sarah Hill, asked what ailed him. He could hardly speak; he answered only, "The feaver." This response frightened Hill. She had heard there was plague in England, and this stranger certainly looked as if he had it. She "encoraged him the more to goe to goodm. Edmonds House & told him there was a doctor woman might doe him some good." Hill saw the man onto a cart that was heading toward the Edmonds homestead.[45]

When he arrived there, Ann Edmonds refused to take him in. Her husband William loaded the stranger (now barely conscious) into his dung cart and set out for the local constable, Thomas Browne. Browne, as reluctant to come in contact with this frighteningly sick man as anyone else, demanded to know why Edmonds was bringing a stranger to his house. Because, said Goodman Edmonds, the man wasn't known to him or his wife, they didn't want to be liable for the costs of caring for an indigent, and because his disease was so strange they didn't know if he had the plague or was perhaps even bewitched. After one more unsuccessful attempt to convince a local family to take the stranger in, Browne unwillingly did so himself. The young man died shortly thereafter.[46]

At first glance, it seems obvious why nobody wanted to take the young man in. After all, the plague was a dreaded disease. While fear of the plague surely played a part in his tragic fate, the fact that he was a stranger in town was just as important. By excluding him from their house, Doctoress Edmonds and her husband were behaving much like their local courts: they were regulating the access of strangers to their town. Small communities were naturally suspicious of outsiders. In particular, localities feared being saddled with indigent strangers who would become financial burdens. Courts enforced this fear by the well-known means of "warning out." Once a poor outsider was warned, he or she could no longer count on local poor relief. Similarly, William Edmonds told Constable Browne, "I doe not look that I am bound to look after him. . . . I might have kept him a month."[47] That the young man was probably a pauper was doubly significant for Ann Edmonds, who charged fees for her services. The rejection of the stranger by two families was an informal warning out by individuals rather than a town. Ironically, in this case, it was the town, represented by Constable Browne, that ended up with the stranger. Rejecting the sick young man was not pure cruelty but a combination of community and institutional xenophobia, combined with financial and health concerns.[48]

Enforcing community concerns had special importance for female healers. Since they played a role in courtrooms that no other women did, it is natural that they took special care to enforce not only laws but also the values behind those laws. Ann Edmonds's rejection of the ailing stranger maintained her authority as a healer and as a potential officer of the court. Her hard stance against poor outsiders marked her as an upstanding member of the community, one whom the court and the other local authorities could trust.

Their burden of enforcement gave midwives a double role. On the one hand, midwives were the central figures of the women's medical community who could and sometimes did act as advocates for women. On the other hand, their unique legal authority obligated them to be particularly strict in upholding local law and custom, and they did not hesitate to turn on women they thought had crossed the line. One side of this ambiguity created moments of premodern "sisterhood": the midwife testifying to the good character of a woman in a lawsuit, or confirming a servant girl's account of sexual assault. However, the other side of the healer's role was just as dramatic: the relentless interrogation of adulteresses and single mothers at their most vulnerable moment, or the doctoress turning a desperately ill man away from her door. Women of the time recognized this double role and avoided midwives and healers when they had something to hide from official authority. As we saw in chapter 3, the Savory and Davis women did not call midwives when Sarah Savory and Sarah Davis gave birth to their illegitimate children. These women and their kin wanted to deceive the court, and calling midwives would have interfered with their schemes. Thus, they chose to risk travail without a midwife's services.

Despite the fears of some of their clients, midwives and healers did their best to strike a balance between compassion and enforcement. When Sarah Boynton accused Ebenezer Browne of beating her with a ladder, inducing a difficult, premature labor, midwives' testimony weighed heavily in the case. The midwives' medical testimony contradicted Sarah's claim: "Shee had much such a travell as shee had with som other of her children and was safe delivered and the child well in health and she as wel as other women in that condition to our apprehentione." However, since Browne had made a counter-accusation against Goodwife Boynton, claiming that she had provoked the dispute, Goodwife Boynton's character was also a key issue. The midwives, Hannah Hazen and Mary Leighton, gave testimony regarding Sarah Boynton's reputation among the local women: "We say that the woman is a peaceaboe, Quiet, well cariaged Neighbour."[49] As midwives, Hazen and Leighton were uniquely qualified to judge not just Sarah Boynton's medical condition but her character as well. In cases like these, they acted as leaders of the women's community, telling the truth as they saw it about the medical merits of a woman's case, but making sure a losing plaintiff's reputation for rectitude did not suffer.

Even more than the Boynton case, the vignette that opens this chapter exemplifies the skill with which female healers balanced their many obligations. When the unmarried Ann Chase went into labor, Elinor Baily's first duty was to the court: to obtain the name of the child's father with a reasonable degree of certainty. To this end, Baily assumed the role of inquisitor. For the six days that it took for the baby to be born, Goodwife Baily repeated her question: who is the father of this child? When Chase's travail grew more difficult and painful, Baily showed no sympathy: "I often told her that it was likely her paines continued ye longer, because Shee had not spoken ye truth."[50]

Having done her duty as an enforcer, Baily then turned to her role as an advocate for Chase. She dutifully reported to the court Chase's tale of sexual assault, emphatically insisting that it was the truth. She added further support to Ann Chase's story by testifying to her character: "The above sd Elingor saith yt Ann Chase lived with her two yeeres a servant & yt shee never saw any light or unseemly Carriage in all yt time."[51] Even though Elinor Baily had no reason to doubt Chase's word when travail began, her position as a court authority demanded that she conduct a rigorous examination. As soon as that duty was fulfilled, she could turn to her role as compassionate midwife: ensuring that John Allen did his duty by the baby, and that Ann Chase retained at least the shreds of a reputation for modesty.

The midwife's double role illustrates the tension created by her legal and cultural authority. When midwives and healers performed their tasks, they were using authority that otherwise was an exclusive male prerogative. Thus, female healers occupied a special place in the gender hierarchy. They could be more assertive than most women, even in their dealings with men. Unlike the general image of women as vacillating and prone to falsehood, their sworn word brought legal consequences to bear on fornicators, adulterers, and rapists. Healing in general, and midwifery in particular, comprised two of the few ways in which women could wield real power.

This power, and other privileges that healers acquired, made the midwife in some ways a figure of ambiguous gender. Her authoritative position in the courtroom was one that was otherwise exclusively male; her legal roles outside the courtroom—questioning witnesses, recording wills—were also male prerogatives. In England, midwives took on some of the power of the clergy as well—they were the only persons other than ministers who could perform baptisms. A woman healer had a whiff of androgyny about her.[52]

It is no surprise, then, that the midwife-healer was somewhat suspect. There had long been an association between midwives and witchcraft. In the sixteenth century, English midwives applying for licenses were asked, "Whether you know of any who do use charms, sorcery, enchantments, invocations, circles, witchcrafts."[53] Women who occupied anomalous positions of power, such as female landowners, were more vulnerable to accusations.[54] Like women landowners, midwives occupied a position that was usually male. This gender ambiguity, combined with the fear and resentment that would naturally grow from healers' roles as enforcers, combined to make healers and midwives witchcraft suspects. While there is little evidence that midwives and healers were actually accused more often than other women, the dark side of the midwife's cultural authority was its potential supernatural origins.

Given this dangerous aspect to their authority, it is no wonder that midwifery manuals urged practitioners to be ultra-feminine in their demeanor. The ideal midwife "ought . . . to be sober, affable, courteous and chaste; not covetous, nor subject to Passion: but bountiful and compassionate, and her Temper chearful and pleasant."[55] Prescriptions such as these ensured that the midwife remained firmly within the bounds of acceptable female behavior. By emphasizing their own sobriety and the private, feminine nature of their work, midwives remained respectable, reliable, and free from witchcraft accusations.

Because of this delicate position, healers' ability to act as women's advocates was limited by the stronger need to maintain the trust of the court. As in the case of Ann Edmonds, this sometimes meant giving up opportunities to use skills and earn income. A healer had to support both the letter and the spirit of the law. While a sympathetic healer could be the best advocate a woman in trouble could have, there was only so much a healer could do. The first irony of the midwife's authority is that she had to limit her advocacy in order to maintain it.

Not only was the extent of healers' authority limited, but so was its scope. In cases where both male and female healers testified, male physicians gave much more detailed testimony and couched it in language very different from that of their female colleagues. Both the midwife Elinor Baily and the physician John Dole were in attendance when George Carr died without a written will. As we saw earlier, Baily testified to Carr's wish that his children work out their own inheritance, and briefly to his confused mental state, saying only that "he was not at that time in a capacity to make his will or to that purpose." Dole's testimony began, "I judged his nerves to be much affected, both the Braine medula Spinalis and the Nervous parts of the Vaines, & bladder by which the other nervous parts of the body were much distempered, I was frequently with him till his death & according to my best Judgment and his owne words signifying the same he was not capable to Setle his estate."[56] We have seen in other cases that Elinor Baily was an articulate witness and keen observer, but when a case fell outside her cultural jurisdiction, as this one did, she withdrew into the background.

The language of Dole's testimony suggests one reason for this: respect for formal education and the authority of science. Dole used Latin terms that demonstrate both his educational level and his familiarity with the latest anatomical discoveries. Midwives, even the most sophisticated, did not have access to this kind of education. This point is succinctly illustrated by testimony in a 1675 case from the Suffolk County Court. John Garland was appealing the sentence imposed on himself and his wife for fornication before marriage. Their child had been born after only seven months; Garland claimed it was a premature birth. To support his case, he produced a midwife and several women who drew on their own experience in their testimony: "I never saw so litle a childe in my life," testified one. Another said it "was so weakly wee were forst to feed it with a feather," and "it haveing no nayles to our apprehenton upon hand nor foot," it must have come before its time. But John Garland himself chose a different tactic. Like John Dole, he chose authority of science to support his case: "Various physikal bookes . . . saith that Children borne in ye seventh month may be borne Legitimate."[57] Experience with newborn babies was clearly a woman's work, but reading authoritative treatises was clearly a man's.

Men's use of the authority of science is connected to another gender issue. The late seventeenth century saw the beginnings of a systematic movement to exclude women from scientific pursuits, including medicine. Science, long personified as female, was being redefined as inherently masculine and as characterized by traits such as rationality and objectivity. Women's traditional knowledge, such as midwifery and herbal medicine, was also being redefined as unscientific. Until midwifery was reincorporated into medicine in the late eighteenth century, it was not considered science and was thus unworthy of learned consideration. Midwifery would not be interesting to scholarly physicians until the eighteenth century, just as male physicians were making inroads into obstetrics. John Dole could thus make his Latinate pronouncements about the male body with great authority, but it might have been beneath his dignity to comment on a childbirth case. Herein lies the second irony of midwives' courtroom authority: they could be more authoritative than other women only because the knowledge they possessed was less than men's. That is, women healers could take their small measure of masculine authority only when dealing with traditional female lore. It was this "ultra-feminine" nature of the midwife's work that put her in a position to instruct men.[58]

Given these limitations, midwives and healers made good use of their authority. While the ideal New England woman was silent and invisible, the public part played by midwives dramatized the value of women and their roles. When a midwife came to court to testify about the father of an illegitimate baby, she participated in a ritual that affirmed all aspects of New England womanhood. She supported general societal values by condemning the woman and her partner for fornication, yet, more often than not, she also tried to soften the court's view of the mother. She described, publicly and under oath, a positive view of women and femininity.

[6]

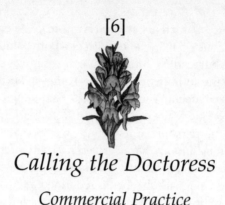

Calling the Doctoress

Commercial Practice

ON A CHILLY MARCH AFTERNOON, Ebenezer Parkman's neighbor Mr. Wood was loading firewood into a cart. As he was standing atop the loaded wagon, the horse shied; he fell under the cart's wheels. The heavy cart passed over his leg, breaking it in two places. Neighbors sent for Mrs. Parker, the local bonesetter. She arrived quickly, bringing her apparatus for pulling bones back into place as well as her splints and bandages. Reverend Parkman comforted his neighbor while Mrs. Parker set the bone. A week later, she returned to check on her patient and change the bandages on his leg.[1]

The courtroom was one place where women healers could exercise authority. Other healers did so by practicing medicine much like male physicians, charging money for their services. In addition to midwives, two kinds of healers collected fees: nurses, and "doctoresses" or "doctor women." Both usually took on chronic or infectious cases, and neither delivered babies. The differences between them started with their level of skill. Nurses were unskilled or semi-skilled—that is, they had no more knowledge of medicine than any ordinary woman. Doctoresses, on the other hand, had special skills—they made medicines, prescribed diets, and dressed wounds.

NURSES

Nurses fit easily into women's practice. Their skills did not differ much from those of housewives. They sat at bedsides, comforted the sick, and administered medicines. Doctoresses, on the other hand, practiced much like midlevel male physicians. These differing styles had very important social effects on their practitioners. Nurses, as one might expect, acted the part of the deferential goodwife. Doctoresses did not, and sometimes paid a price for their autonomy and authority.

Families hired nurses for a number of different tasks. The most common was to care for a woman after childbirth. Usually only affluent women hired an "afternurse" for their lying-in. These nurses relieved the mother of some of her household duties, bathed the baby after birth and brought it to the mother to suckle, and watched at the mother's bedside for any sign of childbed fever or other complications. The nurse Mary Holyoke hired in 1773 had the skill to take care of her patient's minor postpartum complaints. When Holyoke developed a sore breast, the nurse prepared an ointment of parsley, butter, chamomile, and wormwood. Several days later, this same unnamed nurse prepared an emetic medicine for her mistress's upset stomach. Nurses also participated in or suggested folk rituals for the child's well-being, such as laying scarlet cloth on the child's head to protect it from bad air.[2]

Teenage girls sometimes worked as postpartum nurses. This practice served to train young women in infant care and household medicine. Ebenezer Parkman hired his young neighbor Patty Dunlop to look after his wife after several births, noting that "Patty can tend ye Child better yn any one, as she also takes a singular pleasure & Delight in it."[3] Patty's duties also included "waiting on" Hannah Parkman, a description which implies that her position was more that of a maidservant than a medical practitioner.

The term *nurse* could also mean wet nurse. Samuel Sewall noted that the first woman to suckle his eldest son was not his wife but the nurse Bridget Davenport. Some, like Goodwife Parling of Cambridge, Massachusetts, took in orphans or abandoned children. In 1678, she was the only person willing to care for the unfortunate infant born out of wedlock to Hannah Stevenson. Stevenson's father literally left the baby on the doorstep of the house in which its putative father lived. The father refused to take it in. The bewildered constable finally took the child to Goodwife Parling.[4]

A few women offered wet-nursing in addition to their skills in caring for lying-in or sick women. Ruth Williams of Marblehead, Massachusetts, nursed a woman during her fatal bout with childbed fever, then took the infant into her home to suckle. (Unfortunately, when the widowed husband discovered that the child was not his, he stopped paying Williams's fees, forcing her to petition the court for reimbursement.)[5]

While caring for new mothers and infants was the most common job for nurses, there were others. During epidemics, an entire family could fall ill. At these times, some families hired nurses to care for the sick. As with postpartum nurses, their skill level varied. Some of these nurses had great experience. Ann Fox, a mature woman of forty, was hired by the Adams family to nurse them through a smallpox epidemic in 1681. As testimony to her special skills, the Adams family brought her from Boston to their home in Essex County, rather than hire a local woman. Fox set up an isolation ward in the upper chamber of the house for the seven members of the family who fell ill.[6]

Other families hired young girls to nurse them through infectious disease, much as they did for postpartum care. A minor crisis erupted in the Ebenezer Parkman home when several of his children and his wife began to show signs of measles. Hannah Parkman's favorite nurse, Patty Dunlop, was terrified of catching the measles and insisted on being taken home; meanwhile, Ebenezer scoured the neighborhood for a young woman who was willing to take the job. Hannah would not be satisfied with anyone other than Patty Dunlop; even when Ebenezer arrived home with Persis Rice, Hannah pined for Patty, who finally returned.[7] In this case, it seems to have been personal rapport rather than special skills that determined the choice of practitioner.

Nurses also lived with and cared for those who could not care for themselves. In the rare instances where the seriously ill had no relatives capable of looking after them, nurses took the job. Sometimes towns paid their salaries, as when the town of Lynn paid a nurse one shilling to take care of an indigent man and "administer phissick acording to ye docter order."[8] Nurses were also hired to live with the handicapped or frail elderly. Ebenezer Parkman paid a pastoral visit to an elderly, blind parishioner, noting that "Old Mrs. Woods lives with him."[9] In these cases, the nurse's pay was taken from the patient's estate and paid either by a legal guardian or by the executor after the patient's death. Rebeckah Dounton offered her services to the "aged and decrepit, lame and blind" Elinor Robinson, who asked the administrator of her affairs, Mr. Batter, to pay Dounton out of her estate.[10] Probate inventories frequently list nurses as creditors to estates: "to Goodwife Bullocke for fyve days attendance in sickness, 7s 6d"; "to the nurse, 2li, 15s."[11]

Unlike midwives, physicians, and (as we will see shortly) doctoresses, nurses did not do anything beyond what an untrained housewife would do. It was midwives who delivered the babies, diagnosed postpartum complications, and (usually) made decisions about treatment. When the midwife Elizabeth Weeden delivered Samuel Sewall's eldest child, she went about her business expertly, bringing her birth stool and other equipment with her. Afternurses, like Nurse Hurd, served as reliable watchers at the woman's bedside, but their primary duty was to look after the infant during the mother's convalescence.[12]

Nurses had unique opportunities to become intimate with the families they served. They lived with their patients for weeks at a time, which gave them ample chance to participate in bedside scenes and rituals. The care they provided made the sick, the lying-in, and the newborn perhaps more comfortable than they might otherwise have been. In addition to routine tasks like soothing an exhausted mother or walking the floor with a colicky infant, they provided a steady hand and head in more serious situations. They held sick babies in their laps, and if the infant did not recover, they washed and laid out the body. Nurse Hill even helped carry the corpse to the grave when one of the Sewall infants died a few weeks after birth.[13] Such long-term, intimate service led to strong bonds between nurse and patient. As we saw in the case of Patty Dunlop and Hannah Parkman, some women could not be without their favorite nurse any more than they could be without their midwife.

Such family intimacy sometimes led to awkward situations. Isabel Holdred nursed John Chater through a long illness, which gave her ample opportunity to observe Alice Chater's indiscreet behavior with a manservant. Holdred testified that she saw Alice Chater get into the servant's bed, and overheard her tell the servant that she would marry him if her husband's illness proved fatal. Isabel Holdred's work led to even further entanglement with the affairs of the Chater family. A year later, she found herself before the court again—this time presented for "unseemly carriages" with John Chater.[14]

Nurses earned their keep by providing services familiar to every housewife. They became members of the households they served, participating in mourning rituals and soothing or exacerbating family tensions. Nurses were ordinary women, performing ordinary female tasks for pay. Socially, they were part of the gossip, conversation, and squabbles that took place at female bedside gatherings. Culturally, they remained inside women's broadly defined role by doing a housewife's work for patients outside their own family.

DOCTORESSES

Unlike every other kind of female practitioner, doctoresses did not center their care on female medical networks. Doctoresses looked after patients who were not their relatives and often took patients into their own homes. At times, doctoresses stepped in under circumstances where a nurse might also have been engaged. For instance, Anna Brigham of Marlborough, Massachusetts, was hired to take care of a "poor sick woman" who had fallen ill while passing through the town on the way to join her husband.[15] In general, however, doctoresses provided very different kinds of care from what either nurses or midwives provided. They rarely took cases related to childbirth, leaving that to the midwives, and they practiced independently, unlike nurses. While nurses did women's work for pay, doctoresses crossed the gender line and practiced like men.

Doctoresses were highly skilled. Their usual patients had chronic, difficult illnesses for which they created medicines, prescribed diets, and provided round-the-clock care. Some even practiced "sorgery," as did one Goodwife Bradstreete of Rowley, Massachusetts, who charged Henry Sewall ten pounds for this and other services in 1656.[16] Similarly, Mistress Hoyt, also of Essex County, Massachusetts, took Thomas Tewksbury into her home in 1674 to cure his "lame hand."[17] Some skilled women shared some characteristics with doctoresses but did not take pay. For instance, Ebenezer Parkman's neighbor Hepzibah Maynard was often called to treat non-childbirth-related matters but did not ask for money in return. However, these unpaid skilled healers were different from those who charged fees. They did not take patients into their homes as many doctoresses did, and there is no evidence that they called themselves "doctoresses," as did paid practitioners.

Like midwives and physicians, doctoresses were recognized as medical authorities in court cases. Rebecca Banfield of Salem, Massachusetts, appeared twice to describe the injuries of assault victims under her care. In 1667, she cared for a woman who died of her injuries, and appeared in court to say, "Yt ye dead woaman had a sore on her sides in her Sickness." Six years later, Banfield testified that Henry Hall had "most payne . . . in his Back and stomack and that he had spitt an abundance of Bloud."[18]

Women had practiced in this way since the Middle Ages. As early as the tenth century, records mention women's medical practice outside of midwifery. In Salerno, Italy, a town widely known as a center of medical expertise, the women were as famous as the men. Between 1273 and 1410, twenty-four women were listed as surgeons in Naples. The practitioner known as Trota, or Trotula, even wrote a famous text on medical practice. From the twelfth century on, however, medical guilds and universities began to systematically exclude women from practice.[19] Despite this exclusion, numerous women worked as "professional" physicians in seventeenth-century England. Women's "natural aptitude in this direction [allowed] them to maintain their position throughout the seventeenth century."[20] Female practitioners were major participants in the medical marketplace of the time, successfully competing with their male counterparts—both learned and lay. Among the many "empirics" denounced by the College of Physicians were a large number of women. It does seem, however, that doctoresses were on the decline in seventeenth-century England.[21]

The two best-documented case studies of doctoresses in New England come from seventeenth-century Massachusetts. Mary Hale, who ran a smallpox hospital in Boston, and Ann Edmonds, who practiced in her home in Lynn, had successful practices. The careers of these women demonstrate that despite—or because of—their success, some female practitioners suffered negative consequences.

Mary Hale was a widow living in Boston during the mid- to late seventeenth century. She began practicing sometime before 1666, when Increase Mather visited a "sick dying man" at her house. At that time she was fifty-eight years old and probably already widowed. She certainly was widowed by 1680, when her name first appears in the court records as the Widow Hale. Caring for the sick appears to have been Hale's way of supporting herself in her widowhood. She took sick people into her house, charging a weekly sum that covered food and linens as well as medicines and doctoring. Her rates were twenty shillings a week for the first three weeks, and ten shillings a week thereafter.[22]

The most complete description of Hale's practice comes from a 1680 court case. A widowed woman, Mistress Gibbs, had hired her slave Zanckey out to the John Wing household. When Zanckey became too sick to work, a dispute arose concerning his medical bills and the money the Wings still owed on his hire. Mary Hale took care of Zanckey during the acute stages of his illness and was therefore an important witness in the case.[23]

Hale's practice was built around noxious and contagious diseases, primarily smallpox. Smallpox was the original diagnosis in Zanckey and the one that caused the Wings to send him to Widow Hale's. Hale testified that the other patients in her home at the time of Zanckey's illness were smallpox patients. Even given the limited knowledge of how disease spread, plagues like smallpox were of concern to public officials, and quarantine hospitals were common. Mary Hale's house was one place where contagious patients could be looked after.[24]

Hale's fee structure implies that she cared for people with chronic diseases as well. Any disease that was contagious or chronic was reason enough to send the patient to Widow Hale's house, to be cared for without fear of burdening or endangering the rest of the family. This fear was one of the reasons why the Wings kept Zanckey at Hale's even after it became clear that his disease was not smallpox but syphilis.[25]

Another reason may have been both the nature of Zanckey's disease and his position in the Wing household. Syphilis was a shameful disease. Not only was it noxious and disfiguring, but also it was associated with sexual transgression. Furthermore, Zanckey was an African slave. In the Wing house, he no doubt was at the bottom of the household hierarchy—assigned the dirtiest work, bedded in the worst accommodations, and fed the least-appetizing food. When he turned up with a sexual disease, the Wings probably wanted to be rid of him and therefore sent him to the Widow Hale's to be cured.

Hale was also sensitive to the nature of Zanckey's disease. He was only one of many patients at her house that spring. Hale asked the Wings to take Zanckey back when other patients began to complain that he was too "noisome" to bear. The Wings, however, were equally unhappy about Zanckey's condition. Hannah Mann, a servant in the Wing household, testified that the poor man "grew Intollerabell ofensif to the holl famely so that we colld scars Indure the room where he was."[26] Mr. Wing enlisted the aid of the "townesmen of Boston" to convince Hale to keep Zanckey at her house. Hale was reluctant to take Zanckey back at first—after all, he was so "ofensif" he might drive away other paying customers. After some persuasion, Hale agreed.[27]

Hale had a cordial relationship with male practitioners. Two physicians were involved in the Zanckey case: Dr. Hawkins and Dr. Betellor. Both worked cooperatively with Hale. Hale called in Betellor when she realized that Zanckey's disease was more than an ordinary case of smallpox, and Betellor applied an ointment to Zanckey's skin lesions. Dr. Hawkins was one of those who came to persuade Hale to keep Zanckey in her house when he became too much trouble for the Wings. After Hale agreed to care for Zanckey, Hawkins undertook to cure Zanckey's syphilis with a series of purges. Hawkins was a regular visitor at Hale's house while he supervised the cure. Neither Hawkins nor Betellor seemed to see Hale as a threatening competitor—their attitude toward her was that of respect for a fellow practitioner, albeit a lesser one. Indeed, the fact that Hale agreed to have in her house a slave with syphilis implies that she was a low-level practitioner, one who would take patients that more fastidious colleagues would refuse.[28]

Perhaps because of her acceptance of lesser status, Hale was lucky in her relationship with her male colleagues. As we will see shortly, not all doctoresses had such an easy time. Hale was also lucky in collecting her debts—the Wings promptly paid the five pounds they owed for Zanckey's care. Other practitioners had more trouble. Mary Folsham had to sue Robert Rose to extract the money he owed her for "curing his lad" in 1674.[29] But the most spectacular debt case, and the one which best illustrates the tensions that could arise between doctoresses and physicians, was a 1660 case from Lynn, Massachusetts. The testimony in this case provides the most detailed picture we have of a doctoress's practice. It illustrates the kinds of cases taken and methods of treatment, as well as the disputes that could arise with both patients and competing male practitioners.

Ann Edmonds kept an inn with her husband William. Like Mary Hale, Ann Edmonds took patients into her home—a home that, in this case, was uniquely set up to take paying guests. Unlike Hale, Edmonds did not specialize in one kind of patient care. From the scant documentation of her practice that remains, it seems that she was more of a general practitioner, taking difficult cases of all kinds.[30]

William Edmonds sued Henry Green when Green refused to pay for Ann Edmonds's treatment of his daughter Mary. Mary Green's case was indeed difficult. Her father had taken her to at least two other practitioners before consulting Edmonds about her chronically infected leg. One witness described Mary's leg as "running and raw with corruption, swelling and looking eager and red."[31] The Edmonds's son Joseph reported that Mary "had a verie greevious leg as if the flesh were Rotten and it stunke."[32] Some of the flesh had come away, leaving the bone exposed. Ann Edmonds diagnosed the trouble as "king's evil," or tuberculosis of the lymph nodes; the infection may well have been a tubercular infection of the bone.[33]

For the cure of this debilitating illness, Henry Green promised a valuable horse—a "mare colt" of "his own mare's breed." Estimates of the horse's value ranged from nine to fourteen pounds—in any case, this was a very large amount of money. If Edmonds failed to cure his daughter, Green agreed to pay for Mary's food and other living expenses with a cow. Edmonds's fee in this case implies that she was a well-regarded practitioner with enough community confidence to charge high prices and collect them. In fact, when the case went to court, Edmonds was suing not only for the horse she had been promised but also for a total of twenty pounds.[34]

Edmonds worked hard for her money. She kept Mary Green in her house for eleven months. She designed a regimen for her patient that included a special diet and elaborate dressings and poultices for the ulcer on Mary's leg. Edmonds's son Joseph testified that his mother washed and bandaged the sore "with much tenderness" every day, even though the stench was so bad that Joseph could not bear to be in the same room. Edmonds also made sure that the girl ate well, insisting on fresh meat and greens, even in midwinter when the rest of the family made do with salt pork and dried peas.[35]

When these methods failed, Edmonds helped Mary remove a piece of rotten bone from her own leg. A neighbor described the scene:

> I saw ye bone end stand out of her leg about an Inch and after
> that two inches or more and after that . . . ye Childe toulde

mee now the bone is out of my leg and ggd Wife Edmands
fecht the bone to mee it Was six Inches long or more to my
apprehnsion.[36]

Removing the bone improved Mary's condition to the point where
Edmonds declared her cured. Edmonds was fond of showing the
bone to visitors.

From this case it seems that Edmonds's practice was more sophisticated and skillful than Hale's. Hale nursed patients through smallpox and prepared caudle or other soothing drinks to comfort them.
Edmonds took on cases other physicians had given up, made poultices and dressings of her own devising, and in Mary Green's case,
took the initiative to remove a piece of bone. It was perhaps this extra
level of skill that so irritated her male colleagues. Especially piqued
was Thomas Starr, a Charlestown physician who had cared for Mary
Green immediately before her father brought her to Edmonds. When
he heard from a mutual acquaintance that Mary was cured, he refused
to believe it and spluttered that "Hee would eat a firebrand if she
cuered itt."[37] Starr was probably reduced to such statements when
witnesses familiar with both practitioners compared him unfavorably
with Edmonds. One such witness noted that when Mary left Starr,
her leg had a "very bade and di[s]prate wound," but when the witness saw the girl at the Edmonds household she could "goe & Leape
about very Livfly, at which this deponant did much rejoyce at the
good sucsese."[38]

Henry Green produced other witnesses who disputed the cure.
Several of his witnesses were medical practitioners of one sort or another. Dr. Anthony Crosbee examined the girl and sniffed, "according to my best skill I aprehended that the bone was not suficiently
Sealed."[39] Along with the physicians Starr and Crosbee, Green sum-
moned the husband of another doctor woman to testify that the girl's
leg was "no better than it was when she went from my wife . . . not
cured."[40] While calling medical witnesses in a court case like this was
logical, the tone of their testimony suggests that they resented the
competition Edmonds represented and used their testimony to dis-
parage her abilities. In this context, it is also significant that Green and
the witnesses found nothing strange in consulting a variety of practitioners, both male and female. Competition from women may have
been especially annoying, but it was not unusual.

While fellow practitioners did not support Edmonds's efforts, her neighbors did. Sarah Jenkens testified that when Mary Green first came into the Edmonds household, her leg ulcer was "a very dangerous sore to my apprehension." After Edmonds removed the piece of bone, Jenkens said she "saw the leg Healed up."[41] Thomas Marshall visited Mary Green at Thomas Starr's house and at Ann Edmonds's. Like Sarah Jenkens, he testified that the girl's leg was in terrible condition when she left the Starrs. At the Edmonds house he "saw the woman take great paines with the child"; a few months later, he noted that "the childs legg . . . was almost well."[42] Edmonds's local reputation was such that her neighbors rallied to her support in this case, and testified eagerly on her behalf.

The nonmedical witnesses who testified against Edmonds may have had their own reasons for doing so. Green's cousin Giles Fifield testified that Mary's leg was still sore when she returned from Edmonds's household. Fifield was from Charlestown. Presumably he knew Thomas Starr and came to his defense much as Sarah Jenkens and Thomas Marshall came to Ann Edmonds's.[43] Overall, the conflicting testimony on Mary's condition was a mix of professional jealousy and local loyalties. Whatever the truth of the matter may have been, the court sided with Green.

Hale's and Edmonds's practices had much in common. They took on a variety of patients and treated men, women, and children alike. Medicine provided both with an income, which was a major if not the sole means of support. More important, Hale and Edmonds practiced with an authority and independence that was unusual among women healers. This authority manifested itself in several ways. They both practiced in their homes, rather than visiting the patient. Practice at home meant that they were more firmly in charge of the patients' care than they might otherwise have been, without interference from family or visitors. While Hale consulted with physicians from time to time and deferred to their judgment, Edmonds practiced in complete independence from other practitioners, formal or informal. Such independence allowed some doctoresses to claim cures as completely their own. One enterprising doctoress, Mrs. Kimball, sold medicines christened with her own name.[44]

Doctoresses were differentiated from other female practitioners by their clientele, their fees, and the social context of their work. Midwives' practices were limited to childbirth-related ailments and women's complaints. Midwives charged so little for their services it seems unlikely that they relied on their midwifery for much of an income. Compare the five shillings midwives charged for a delivery to the ten shillings a doctor woman charged for healing a sore breast, the twenty shillings a week Mary Hale charged her patients, the eight pounds Rebecca Banfield received for caring for a child's broken leg, or the horse worth fourteen pounds promised to Ann Edmonds.[45] The social context of doctoresses' practice also distinguished them from their female colleagues. In the court cases describing Hale's and Edmonds's practices, nowhere is there a mention of the groups of women who normally surrounded sickbeds. Instead, the picture that emerges is that of Hale and Edmonds attending their patients quite alone.

All of these factors came together to make a doctoress's practice much more like that of a male physician than that of any other female healer. As we have seen, Thomas Starr and Ann Edmonds had similar methods and policies toward their patients—caring for patients with chronic diseases in their own homes. Another good comparison with Edmonds's practice is that of Dr. Philip Reade. Reade was an itinerant physician who rode a regular circuit through Massachusetts. His route included towns such as Lynn (where Edmonds lived and worked), Salem, Sudbury, Cambridge, and his own hometown of Concord. Reade usually set up a "clinic" at an inn where he saw patients and dispensed medicines. He had many regular patients drawn from all levels of society, from prosperous farmers to servants and slaves.[46]

As is the case with Edmonds, the best record of Reade's practice is a debt case. Reade treated a young boy in his home much as Ann Edmonds treated Mary Green. He cared for the boy over one winter and provided "diet" as well as "salves and playsters" and several "vomits." Also like Edmonds, Reade was forced to sue to collect his fees. The boy's father claimed that the boy was not cured, and that Reade had kept him far beyond the "month or five weeks" they had originally agreed upon. In fact, the major difference between the Reade and Edmonds lawsuits is that Reade won his case and collected the five pounds, seven shillings owed to him.[47]

All of these factors came together to put doctoresses at the margins of appropriate female behavior. It should not be surprising, then, that doctoresses were more vulnerable than other female healers to accusations of witchcraft. In noting that women practitioners seemed to be accused more often than other women, John Demos wrote, "We cannot discover how many New England women tried their hand at doctoring, but we know that some who did so brought down on themselves a terrible suspicion."[48] It was not the practice of medicine per se that brought about this suspicion, but the way in which some women practiced it. Those accused were women healers who stepped outside the normal boundaries of female practice—by practicing for money, by taking non-childbirth-related cases, and by not being part of the women's medical community. Both Ann Edmonds and Mary Hale were accused of witchcraft. The two cases bear close examination.

Hale was accused of witchcraft in 1681 by a young man named Michael Smith, a boarder in her house. She apparently had some hopes that Smith would marry her granddaughter, but Smith was courting another woman, Margaret Ellis. According to Ellis's testimony, when Hale discovered Smith's marital intentions, she fell into a rage and swore that Ellis "should never Enjoy him after." Smith tried to appease Hale by drinking a cup of ale with her, but shortly afterward, he fell violently ill.[49]

Understandably, Smith did not want to consult Hale about his illness. He went to the house of the widow Hannah Weacome, telling her that "Guddy Haile had bewitched him." While not identified as such, Weacome, it seems, was another practitioner—perhaps of the kind known in England as a cunning woman, one who mixed magic with medical practice. Weacome put Smith to bed in her house and performed a ritual designed to find the witch who was tormenting Smith. She put some of his urine in a bottle and corked it. Soon, Mary Hale appeared at the door and "did not seace walking to and froo, about the House." She continued for about an hour, until the other women at Weacome's house persuaded Weacome to uncork the bottle, whereupon Hale went home.[50]

Perhaps as a peace gesture, Hale made a caudle for Smith and sent it to him as he lay at Widow Weacome's. Smith refused to accept it. Margaret Ellis, who seemed to be skeptical of Smith's accusation, led him to believe that she had made it herself and persuaded Smith to drink it. That night, Smith had a terrible nightmare, groaning in his sleep so much that Ellis thought, "Ye walls of ye house would have falleun on us." When Smith awoke, he called for Hale's immediate arrest, saying that Goodwife Hale had appeared to him and taken him to a witch's banquet.[51]

This case makes a subtle but clear connection between Smith's accusation and Hale's medical practice. Smith had been a boarder at Hale's house and must have been aware of her extensive medical practice. The events in this case took place only a year after the Zanckey incident, so it is possible that Smith had witnessed Hale's care of Zanckey and the smallpox patients. In this context, it becomes significant that the effect Hale's supposed witchcraft had on Smith was to make him sick. Furthermore, at least part of the means by which Smith claimed Hale had bewitched him was associated with her care of the sick—the caudle she sent after he fell ill.

It is also significant in this context that one of the witnesses supporting Smith's claim was another female healer. Weacome took sick people in as boarders, just as Hale did. Perhaps she saw Smith's illness as a way of eliminating a competitor. What is more interesting is the evidence that Weacome, unlike Hale, was a full member of the women's medical community. A group of women had gathered at Smith's sickbed and witnessed Weacome's counterspell—it was these very women who asked Smith to uncork the bottle and let Hale go home. Margaret Ellis came to Weacome's to help nurse Smith, anticipating her role as his wife.

Indeed, the entire case against Hale stemmed from a dispute over women's business, over which woman was to marry Michael Smith. When this dispute between women became a witchcraft case, it was the woman who was the farthest outside the women's community who became the target. Just as midwives and other healers could protect other women in court cases, it seems that membership in the women's medical community provided some shelter from witchcraft accusations. Hannah Weacome openly practiced magic, and there is no evidence that Hale ever did so. Yet it was Hale who found herself in court, in a case connected to her medical practice. The case against Hale was not strong enough for the jurors, however; her trial ended in an acquittal.

Ann Edmonds also found herself accused of witchcraft. The surviving details of the accusation provide enough tantalizing hints to be cause for speculation and not much more. However, the few facts that remain suggest that her case, too, began as a dispute over women's business and was directly connected to her medical practice.

The surviving record of the Edmonds case is the decision by the Court of Assistants to dismiss the charges. The court "saw no Ground to fix any charge against her." The complaint had been brought by the Edmondses' neighbors Samuel Bennett and his wife, and the Bennetts were ordered to pay the Edmondses' travel expenses and witness fees. Immediately following the Edmonds case on the same page is a court decision regarding the Bennetts. Samuel and Sarah Bennett, and Samuel's brother John, were bound over to appear at the Court of Assistants along with the maidservant Elinor Squire. The four of them were to answer for the "great neglect of Alice Wilson," which had left her at the point of death, and more suggestively, "for burying [Wilson's] child in an obscure and clandestine manner in the garden of the said Samuel Bennett." The Bennetts were ordered to pay forty-six shillings for Alice Wilson's "phisick, diet, etc.," as well as "Wm. Edmonds and Anna Edmonds their witnesses and charges, which comes to thirty-two shillings."[52]

What happened here? It is hard not to infer that the two cases are connected—that the accusation of Ann Edmonds was connected to the illness of Alice Wilson and the death of her child. Did Edmonds try to heal Wilson and fail? A more sinister possibility is that an infanticide or botched abortion had taken place, and Edmonds was involved. In this case, it is possible that the Bennett women accused Edmonds before she accused them.

Given that the Bennett–Wilson case involved a woman and her child, it seems likely that whatever happened to Alice Wilson was a gynecological or obstetrical case—the kind of case that normally would have been taken care of by a midwife and a group of women. Ann Edmonds was not an active participant in such gatherings. Did Edmonds intrude where she was not wanted, or when things went terribly wrong, did the Bennett women decide to blame the healer most alien to them—the one who was on the far edge of the women's circle?

We may never know the answers to these questions in Ann Edmonds's case. However, another, better-documented, witchcraft case has themes similar to that of the Bennett–Wilson case. In this example, a woman with a reputation as a healer was deliberately excluded from a childbirth gathering. The outcome became a piece of evidence in the witchcraft case against her.

Elizabeth Morse was accused of witchcraft after a long and complicated case that involved her grandson and a young male boarder.

Suspicion fell first on the boarder but landed at last on Morse. Eventually, she was convicted and sentenced to death. Testimony in her trial implied that prior to her accusation Morse had done some healing among her neighbors—though how formally or whether or not she was paid is unclear. After the whisperings of witchcraft began, her healing skills came back to haunt her. In an echo of the Mary Hale case, many of those who accused Morse complained of strange illnesses and physical symptoms, ranging from the mundane (bloody flux) to the bizarre ("one of [her breasts] rotted away from her"). She was also accused of killing a child by stroking its head when it was sick.[53]

Even before the accusations began, some of her neighbors refused to have her near them when they fell ill. The incident that most resonates with the Edmonds witchcraft case started when a neighbor woman went into labor. The woman was fearful of inviting Morse, since the rumors of witchcraft had already begun, but as her labor "continued a long season" with no sign of the child, the women attending her urged her to invite Goodwife Morse. Morse was reluctant to come at first, but at last was convinced. Soon after Morse arrived, the child was born. Despite the positive outcome of the case, this incident was proffered as evidence of the supernatural origins of Morse's healing skill. The witness stated that Morse had been insulted by not being called. Morse must have impeded her neighbor's labor until she was sent for, then, her feelings being assuaged, she allowed it to proceed.[54]

Perhaps the situation that led to the death of Alice Wilson's child was similar: a local female healer, an outsider to the women's community, called in to a difficult case at the last minute. In Edmonds's case, probably the negative outcome of the medical problem led directly to the witchcraft accusation, while in Morse's the childbed episode was only one incident among many that brought her before the court. Both cases share one key element, however—a woman healer who was not part of the women's community, for whatever reason.

Dr. Philip Reade, whose debt case so resembled Ann Edmonds's, was also familiar with the courtrooms of both Middlesex and Essex Counties. However, his legal history provides an instructive contrast with those of Hale, Edmonds, and Morse. When Reade was in court, he was usually plaintiff rather than defendant. He used the law to challenge competing practitioners and dissatisfied patients alike. Unlike his female peers, Reade had nothing to fear from exercising autonomy and authority in his medical practice. Rather than be on the defensive, he used his suits to assert his authority and defend his professional reputation.

This assertiveness was typical of Reade's personal style—indeed, many of the documents that mention him describe an aggressive, even abrasive personality. His sharp tongue often led to trouble; in one incident, Reade exploded at his pious mother-in-law, "The divill take you and your prayers." This comment landed him in court for blasphemy. Nor was this the only time Reade suffered the consequences of his temper. One of his ex-patients claimed Reade had "given him such language that hee would not bear it" and threatened to "get a stick and . . . knok out the Doktor's brains."[55]

Reade did not hesitate to sue for slander when his professional competence was questioned. In 1669, he slapped Martha Hill with a one-hundred-pound slander suit when she was rumored to say that Reade "had Cured Sara Wyman of a Swelling under her chin and another under her Apron." The first recipient of this gossip was, interestingly, a woman named Goodwife Blood, a midwife. When Martha Hill first heard the rumor, she went straight to a woman healer with the news. Given Reade's position in the competitive medical marketplace, this fact must have rankled him. In fact, Reade made a point of specifically mentioning Blood's vocation in his slander complaint against Hill. Reade must have feared that a reputation for shady dealings and quackery would quickly follow on the heels of this rumor, and filed suit to stop it in its tracks.[56]

Reade's sensitivity concerning his reputation and to the threat presented by women healers may explain his active participation in witchcraft cases. In 1669, he was one of the principal witnesses against a woman healer named Ann Burt. Burt was a widow living in Lynn, Massachusetts. The witchcraft case is the only documentation of her healing practice; from the evidence presented in court, it would seem that she made medicines, diagnosed illness, and may have also taken patients into her home. Disgruntled patients testifying against her mentioned that she provided care or medicines for headaches and sore throats. Reade's involvement came about when two young women who had been under Burt's care fell into the familiar "fits" associated with witchcraft. Reade examined the two women and "did plainly perceive that there was no natural cause for such unnatural fits." He then began to quiz one of his patients about the agency behind her affliction: "One hour after she had a sadder fit than ever she had afore: then I asked her who afflicts her now." The answer was Ann Burt.[57]

No record remains of a formal witchcraft trial for Burt. Four years after the accusations were made, she died in her own bed, so it would seem that either the charges were dismissed or she was acquitted.[58] Given Reade's abrasive personality and fragile ego, it is plausible that he did in fact see women like Burt as dangerous competitors, and seized the opportunity to eliminate them. Just as Hannah Weacome used her "cunning" skills to mark a competing healer as a witch, Philip Reade used his medical expertise to do the same.

Reade's participation in witchcraft trials raises another gender issue. Reade was able to continue his successful practice in spite of his sharp tongue and unpleasant personality. Evidence suggests that a woman healer in similar circumstances would not have been as fortunate. Men had much more leeway to be disruptive, to brawl with their neighbors, and to curse their enemies. A woman with such a manner would often find herself suspected of witchcraft, while a man would be fined for assault or bound to good behavior for cursing. Reade's behavior both in and out of court demonstrates the considerable freedom he had to actively assert his rights and demand the respect to which he believed he was entitled. Neither Hale nor Edmonds could exercise similar freedom.[59]

When a woman behaved like a man—practiced independently, brought in an income, competed with male practitioners, and most important, practiced outside the women's community—she opened herself up to attack. The attacks came as much from other women like Hannah Weacome as from protoprofessional men like Reade. An independent, authoritative woman was anomalous and therefore dangerous, especially to other female healers. The ambivalence toward women's authority and autonomy in early New England created a cultural association between female healers and witchcraft. Hanging over the head of every female practitioner was the threat, if not the reality, of a witchcraft accusation. Hannah Weacome knew this, and it is possible that her attack on Mary Hale served to deflect suspicion from herself. Philip Reade, for all his slander suits and threats of violence, never had to face this possibility.

Despite this threat, witchcraft accusations were not an inevitable consequence of women's healing practice, even of doctoresses' practice. Of the 104 witchcraft cases John Demos found in New England between 1638 and 1697 (excluding Salem), only 13 involved a woman known to be a healer.[60] Yet it is also true that some women healers were accused. Those who were fell into two categories—women like Elizabeth Morse who had reputations for witchery that went beyond their medical practices; and those, like Ann Edmonds and Mary Hale, whose practices put them in anomalous gender positions. The deciding factor in the outcome of these cases was the woman's previous reputation for witchcraft. Those who had been followed by rumors for a long time were convicted; those whose reputations were otherwise clean were acquitted or never went to trial.[61]

Indeed, some accused healers, such as Winifred Holman and her daughter Mary, successfully sued their accusers for slander. In their case, a neighbor accused the two of them of bewitching his daughter and grandchild. In the winter of 1659, John Gibson confronted Winifred Holman about her hens eating his corn. Shortly thereafter, Gibson's married daughter, Rebecca Stearns, began to suffer from mysterious fits. Both Holman women offered medical advice, and Winifred Holman offered "some herbs . . . that she should use." Rebecca Stearns's fits only worsened, and in addition, her child "fell away in the lower parts." Once again, Mary Holman offered her help, this time for the child, whose ailment she diagnosed as rickets. The Stearnses refused the Holmans' help, but both Rebecca's fits and the child's lameness grew worse—eventually the child's legs wasted away so that the child could not walk, and the spine grew crooked. On this evidence, the Stearnses and the Gibsons had the Holmans arrested. A grand jury was not convinced, however, and refused to issue an indictment.[62]

Soon thereafter, the Holmans successfully sued John Gibson for slander. He was ordered to apologize and was fined. Despite the Gibsons' and Stearnses' damning testimony, no one else stepped forward to accuse the Holmans. Clearly, they were respected and well liked in their community, and they had no previous reputation for witchcraft. Another reference to Winifred Holman in the Middlesex County court records underlines her conventionality: she petitioned to have one of her other daughters, Elizabeth, removed from the service of a man who had "turned to ye accursed sick[ness] of the Quakers forsaking ye Holy ordinances of God Whereby the mortall soul of Her sd. child is endangered."[63]

Perhaps more significantly, the Holmans were also respected members of the Cambridge community. Their neighbors, men and women alike, supported them rather than their accusers. Twenty-five of Winifred Holman's neighbors signed a deposition stating that "we have not any grounds or reason to suspect her for witchery."[64]

While cases like that of the Holmans illustrate that many doctoresses had the support of their neighbors, they should not obscure the fact that some healers were vulnerable. In the Holmans' case, this vulnerability is demonstrated by the fact that they were accused at all. It was their medical practice that distinguished these otherwise respectable women from the rest of their neighbors, and that made them suspicious in the eyes of their accusers. Doctoresses were the most likely of all healers to be targeted for witchcraft accusations, since they, unlike all other women healers, ventured into general practice and transgressed the boundaries of women's healing. Other paid practitioners such as midwives and nurses were central members of female medical networks and kept their practices part of women's traditional work. Hence, nurses, whose practice superficially resembled that of doctoresses, were relatively safe, while doctoresses were not.

Doctoresses' practice slowly declined over the course of the seventeenth century. By the time of the Revolution, few women called themselves doctoresses, even though some still supported themselves as informal practitioners or as midwives. Despite this decline, women never really stopped practicing medicine. Instead, as gender definitions and medical practice changed, so did the definition of female healers.

Epilogue

The Changing Context of the Healer's Calling

IN LATE AUGUST 1752, Hannah Parkman was preparing her still. Her husband had been sick for almost a month, with fever, night sweats, faintness, and pain and swelling in his joints. He had not had much of an appetite for most of that time and had become disturbingly thin. The Parkmans consulted a physician, Dr. Scannell, who taught Hannah to make the medicine her husband needed, a combination of meat, roots, and herbs run through the still. The neighborhood women would come later in the day to watch at Ebenezer's bedside, tend to his needs, and feed him spoonfuls of the cordial she was about to make. Hannah was grateful to them for their help, but she was even more grateful that she had gotten the advice of a learned physician who had studied the latest methods from London.[1]

The Parkmans lived during the eighteenth century, a time of great cultural change in the New England colonies. The colonies had developed a much closer relationship with England, and the two societies gradually became more alike, intellectually, economically, and socially. Such changes affected medicine and medical practitioners. Male physicians in particular began to view themselves as part of an international scientific community—as cosmopolitan professionals, rather than provincial craftsmen. This new self-definition for doctors took place at the same time as subtle changes in gender roles. Paid work, law, and commerce were increasingly walled off as exclusively male territory. Women's roles, whether as housewives, mothers, or medical practitioners, became more restricted as a result. While women were still practicing medicine, and would continue to do so through the eighteenth century and into the nineteenth, the nature of their practice changed.

As we have seen, male and female healers often worked together cooperatively. While women generally deferred to men's knowledge and expertise, they both worked in an atmosphere of mutual respect. In the mid-eighteenth century, however, changes in medicine, gender expectations, and the distribution of ideas began to affect this relationship. As the port cities grew and became more cosmopolitan, the latest European medical knowledge became more accessible and more widely distributed. More male practitioners were able to earn European degrees. The nascent medical societies encouraged uneducated male practitioners to attend their lectures and use their libraries, but they excluded women. Physicians' new self-definition precluded the collegiality that had existed between male and female practitioners in the past. In addition, patients were impressed with the new medical knowledge coming from Europe and were much quicker to call on male physicians than they had been in the past.

Changes in medicine coincided with subtle alterations in gender ideologies and the definitions of public and private life. As the formal public structures—that is, the courts and business, especially long-distance commerce—gained in political power and social prestige, the informal public structures of women's social and economic lives lost influence. Indeed, women's work—whether domestic production of foodstuffs, informal barter, or medical practice—was increasingly defined as belonging solely to the private realm of the household and family. The influence that women's medical networks had in the seventeenth century began to fade. Meanwhile, male social networks assumed a new importance in the social context of medicine as well as in trade, law, and politics.[2]

By the time of the Revolution, male practitioners would be much more (but not completely) dominant. Male physicians became the practitioners of first, rather than last, resort, even in cases concerning female reproductive maladies. As the century progressed, women gradually took on a secondary, supportive role. Women's medical practice, once such a crucial part of public life, was redefined as part of private and domestic life. With the important exception of midwives, local female healers lost respect, prestige, and patients to male physicians.

Male physicians were also redefined. Elite male practice became the model for all types of medicine. Doctors were now part of a self-conscious professional community, and scientific advances in medicine were such that this model of healing had an inherent appeal for patients as well. More and more, patients—male and female, rich, poor, and middling—chose male doctors as their primary practitioners.

Even in this new context, much of women's medical practice remained the same. They continued to do much of the daily work of medicine. Midwives still had a virtual monopoly on care during childbirth, especially in rural areas, and women still did most of the day-to-day work of caring for the sick. Healing also remained deeply embedded in the social networks of a community. Women continued to gather at bedsides, and patients continued to rely on the comfort of female sickbed rituals, even as they sought the perceived benefits of male-dominated medicine. Thus, while change was in the air, it coexisted with continuity and proceeded at a decidedly uneven pace.

Ebenezer Parkman's diary is a detailed record of both the changes and the continuities in the social aspects of medical practice. Over the sixty-four years Parkman kept his journal, he and his large family consulted numerous practitioners, from local doctor women to academically trained physicians. His diary documents a gradual shift in his family's attitude toward medical care. The vignette that opens this chapter depicts a moment in the transition: a housewife makes a medicine, but one that was prescribed by an educated male physician; a group of women come to the house to nurse a sick man, but only after a doctor had been there first. The Parkman diary illustrates both the continuing importance of female medical practice and the increasing patient preference for educated male physicians.

One reason for the changes in the Parkman family experience is simple: there were more male doctors available to consult. Even in the rural village of Westborough, there were so many physicians that Parkman told one young doctor, "I can't recom'd this place for him to settle in."[3] Parkman's perception is borne out by statistics. Between 1700 and 1790, the number of elite physicians grew faster than the general population. During this period, the population in Massachusetts increased by 24.3 percent every ten years; the number of doctors, by 32.4 percent. By 1780, there was one doctor for every 417 people, more than twice as many as there had been one hundred years earlier.[4]

A situation that arose in April of 1759 illustrates this change. Hannah Parkman fell ill with a fever, and shortly thereafter, two of the children followed suit. Ebenezer promptly sent for not one but three doctors: Dr. Chase, Dr. Crosby, and Dr. Willis. Dr. Crosby diagnosed Hannah with "fever and ague" and the children with measles. Dr. Willis prescribed a strong emetic for Hannah, which made her vomit sixteen times, until she was forced to admit "she thinks it will be too hard for her." Dr. Crosby promptly modified the prescription.[5]

The Parkmans' increasing use of male physicians reflects the growing availability of academic medical knowledge and its appeal to patients. The doctors of Westborough probably had not earned European medical degrees, but the emerging medical science that characterized eighteenth-century Europe was slowly making its way to the colonies. Academic medicine had always carried a certain cachet with patients. Practitioners and patients alike were eager to use the new discoveries.

The first medical school in British North America was founded in Philadelphia in 1765. The curriculum was based on that of the prestigious medical school of the University of Edinburgh. Significantly, it included basic science courses such as chemistry, mineralogy, and botany, as well as anatomy and pharmaceutics. The professors were men who had European degrees and who were eager to institute medical science in America. Over the next twenty years, physicians in New York and Boston would do the same, firmly establishing academic medicine in the United States.[6]

The availability of such an education on home soil created a demand for credentialed professionals. At about the same time as the establishment of medical schools, physicians in the major cities founded medical societies. At first, the societies emulated the European model, limiting and regulating the number of physicians through very strict licensing requirements. The Boston society eventually reduced its licensing requirements to merely taking and passing an examination. It assisted those interested in taking the exam by opening their lectures and demonstrations to any "gentleman" who wished to attend. As a result, the number of licensed physicians increased substantially, and patients could assume that a doctor with a license from the society had at least a modicum of scientific knowledge.[7]

Changes in medical practice paralleled changes in broader male social and professional networks. In the eighteenth century, men of all walks of life began to use kin and social networks to extend their commercial and professional reach. In the case of the Parkmans, one of the first male doctors to attend the family on a regular basis was a relative: Hannah Parkman's brother-in-law, Benjamin Gott. Gott was regarded as "a learned and useful Physician and Surgeon" who was "a lover of Learning and learned Men."[8]

Gott's name first turns up in Ebenezer Parkman's diary in 1728, where he is mentioned as a guest in the Parkman's home. For the first ten years of their acquaintance, Gott appears to be solely a relative and friend, not a medical practitioner. He was instrumental in forwarding Parkman's courtship of his wife's sister, Hannah Breck, who would soon become Parkman's second wife. On March 19, 1737, Parkman wrote in his diary, "a.m. to Dr. Gott's, but a short space with Mrs. Hannah." Six months later, Hannah Breck and Ebenezer Parkman married.[9] Even after their marriage, the couple did not use Gott's services immediately. Hannah Parkman suffered a miscarriage in February of 1738, but Dr. Gott is not mentioned in the diary. Instead, Hannah was attended by female kin. Benjamin Gott continued as a regular guest in the Parkman household but did not provide medical services. The first mention of Gott in a medical context occurred in July of 1738, when Parkman brought Gott with him to visit a sick parishioner.[10]

This visit marked a turning point in the Parkmans' relationship with Gott. Only a month later, Parkman sent his oldest son, Ebenezer Jr., to Gott for evaluation of a "swelling in his neck." After that, Gott became a regular attendant to the Parkman family.[11]

The next time Hannah Parkman had a problem pregnancy, Dr. Gott was there. She "swell'd greatly in her Limbs" and was "full of Pain." While a group of women, including the local midwife, had been watching with Hannah for several days, Ebenezer sent for Dr. Gott as soon as the situation became critical. Indeed, Parkman noted that the midwife and other women were "visiting" with Hannah, but he did not mention that his wife was ill until he decided to send for Dr. Gott. Although Parkman did not record what Gott did for Hannah, Gott spent two days with the Parkmans. Eventually, Hannah gave birth to a weak, premature infant. Midwife Granny Forbush and the usual group of women, including Hannah's sister, Dr. Gott's wife, were in attendance.[12]

At the same time that the Parkmans started using Gott's medical services, his social visits to the Parkman household also increased—

in part, no doubt, because of the new family tie. During the first ten years of Parkman's acquaintance with Gott, Parkman recorded only six visits with him. After he married Hannah Breck, the social visits increased along with the medical visits. Gott and Parkman saw each other socially five times in 1738 alone and four times the following year.[13]

The medical relationship and the social ties between Gott and the Parkmans grew in parallel. Medical practice was an economic relationship as well as a personal one. Men's trading partnerships were often based on kin ties and other personal contacts. Similarly, Gott took advantage of his ties with the Parkmans to expand his practice. The kin tie through Hannah Breck established a relationship that Gott could use for his economic advantage, and in turn Parkman could use it to ensure medical care for his family.[14]

Evidence in the diary suggests that Hannah Breck Parkman usually made the choice to send for male doctors when she or the children were sick. The increasing use of bleeding in the family demonstrates this pattern. Ebenezer recorded no instances of bloodletting at all from the beginning of his journal in 1719 until 1736. Between 1737, when Hannah and Ebenezer married, and 1739, the Parkmans employed a doctor to bleed them six times. Between 1740 and 1770, there are ten descriptions of therapeutic bleeding. Hannah was the usual patient. She was bled for ailments ranging from difficult pregnancies to "pluretic fever."[15] The increase in bleeding after Hannah entered the household, combined with the fact that it was usually she who underwent the procedure, strongly implies that it was Hannah, rather than Ebenezer, who desired the services of male physicians.

Hannah Parkman's choices also reflect the continuities in women's practice. Even as she took the initiative in bringing more male physicians to the Parkman household, she continued to participate in traditional sickbed practices and call women healers to attend her and the children. Women still attended Hannah Parkman in childbirth, and a consistent group of female neighbors and kin regularly came to the house to prepare medicines and "watch" with the sick. Included in this group was Hannah's cousin, Anna Brigham Maynard, who had a reputation as a healer in her own right. The Parkmans consulted Granny Maynard on issues related to routine childbirth; Cousin Anna, for help with sick children; and Mrs. Parker, the local bonesetter, when a neighbor broke his leg.[16]

However, the women played a secondary role in caring for the sick and, in particular, in making medical decisions. Dr. Crosby pronounced the diagnosis, not Hepzibah Maynard. When Dr. Willis suggested and supplied an emetic, Cousin Anna monitored its effects and presumably, cleaned up the mess.[17] Over the years that Ebenezer kept his diary, the Parkmans turned more and more to male practitioners first, even in situations where, years earlier, they had called a woman.

This change is most striking in the case of childbirth and female complaints. In 1725, shortly after the birth of her first child, Ebenezer's first wife Molly developed an abscess in her breast. Ebenezer dutifully sent for the midwife, Mrs. Whitcomb, who "broke," or lanced, the abscess. In 1758, Hannah Parkman underwent an extremely difficult childbirth, attended by both Granny Maynard and Dr. Crosby. After the child was born, Hannah fell ill with a breast infection, much as Molly Parkman had in 1725. However, instead of sending for their neighbor Granny Maynard, who had delivered the child, Hannah Parkman called in Dr. Rice and Dr. Hemingway.[18]

The women who came to attend Hannah played subtly different roles than they had in years past. They offered emotional support and watching, and took charge of the children. There is less evidence that they brought their own herbal medicines or plants from their gardens, as, for instance, Elizabeth Davenport and her peers did. They were less likely to perform minor surgery or other more difficult medical tasks—as when Dr. Rice and Dr. Hemingway came to tend Hannah's infected breast. In short, women were taking a more secondary role as nurturers and supporters, rather than the central role their forebears had played, that of active medical practitioner.

As was the case with bleeding, this change in roles reflected Hannah Parkman's desires, and she was not alone in this. European obstetrical techniques became more common in the colonies, and women who could afford to chose male physicians over the traditional midwife. The male doctors had access to the newest obstetrical technology. One of these technologies, forceps, allowed the extraction of infants that previously could not have been delivered without great injury to the mother, if at all. In addition, physicians could give their patients the only available anesthetic of the time, opium. The perception of greater safety and comfort created by these practices attracted wealthy, urban women away from midwives. As we saw with the Parkmans, similar forces were at work in general medical practice. The chemical medi-

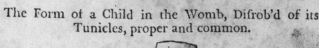

The Form of a Child in the Womb, Difrob'd of its Tunicles, proper and common.

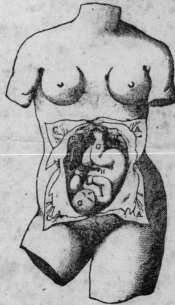

The Explanation of the Figure.

A A THE Portions of the *Chorion*, diffect-ed and removed from its proper place.

B A Portion of the *Amnios*.

CC The Membrane of the Womb diffect-ed.

DD The *Placenta*, being a flefhy Subftance endued with many fmall Veffels, by the which the Infant receives its Nourifhment.

E The Varication of tho Veffels which make up the Navel ftring.

FF The Navel ftring, by which the Umbi-licar Veffels are carried from the *Pla-centa* unto the Navel.

GG The Infant as it lieth perfect in the Womb near the time of Delivery.

H The Infertion of tho Umbilic Veffels in-to the Navel of the Infant.

Pfalm CXXXIX. xiii, xiv, xv, xvi.

To thee, O bleffed LORD, my Voice I'll raife,
And to thy glorious Name aferibe the Praife,
That thou haft me fo wonderfully made,
And in my Mother's Womb in Darknefs laid:
And there thofe Wonders wrought'ft no tongue can tell;
Thy Works are Marvellous, I know right well:
My Subftance was not hid from thee, when I
Within the Womb was wrought fo curioufly:
And my unfinifh'd Parts were all furvey'd
By thee, and thoroughly fafhioned or made.

Plate from *Aristotle's Compleat Masterpiece*. This popular medical manual, which went through multiple editions in both England and America, was aimed specifically at midwives. This plate from a mid-eighteenth-century edition demonstrates how scientific knowledge was disseminated to an audience of female healers. (Yale University, Harvey Cushing/John Hay Whitney Medical Library.)

cines and bleeding Hannah Parkman desired were available only from male doctors. Although Parkman continued to employ a midwife for her lying-ins, she was much quicker to call a male physician than her mother would have been.[19]

Female practitioners themselves were eager to take advantage of the new knowledge and practices. Richard Brown noted that midwives and other healers were more than willing to learn from their "betters" and did so through personal instruction from elite male physicians and popular medical books. Indeed, by 1726, printed home medical manuals were widely available, and women were using them. In that year, Sarah Walker and her husband bought a copy of *The Husbandman's Guide* (which included culinary and veterinary recipes as well as medicines for curing human illness) and inscribed it with her name and a record of the births of their children.[20]

The increasing availability of academic medical knowledge is reflected in the nature and quantity of medical books sold in New England. In the seventeenth century, most of the books for sale came from the estates of learned men, usually ministers. The medical books in these sales were almost always in foreign languages, especially Latin, but also Italian, French, and Greek. Such books were obviously intended for a limited, elite audience. As the eighteenth century opened, booksellers began to import new books directly from London. More titles were available in English, and copies of popular books such as *Digby's Closet* (a compendium of herbal remedies that went through numerous editions during the seventeenth and eighteenth centuries) started to appear among the scholarly treatises such as *Mr. Watson's Essay on Fevers, the Rattles and Canker*. On the eve of the Revolution, the books available proliferated. The works were now primarily in English, and popular home health guides made up almost half of the inventory for one book sale held in Boston.[21]

The Parkman diary records an example of the effect these newly available books had on women practitioners. In 1760, Ebenezer Parkman gave Anna Brigham Maynard a copy of a pamphlet on the treatment of smallpox he had purchased on one of his trips to Cambridge. Maynard eagerly accepted the pamphlet, written by Dr. Nathaniel Williams and entitled *The Method of Practice in the Small-Pox with Observations on the way of Inoculation*.[22] When Ebenezer purchased the book, he was doing a kindness for a relative, but he was also changing the way his cousin the doctoress practiced her craft.

The pamphlet itself reflects many of the changes in eighteenth-century medicine. It begins with a recitation of the credentials of the author: "He had his Education at Harvard College and studied Chymistry and Physick." Later, it states that "he has consulted with Dr. Mead and other principal Physicians in England for Advice and Help." Scientific education and European connections were primary in establishing the legitimacy of the author and his advice.[23]

Further, the stated purpose of the pamphlet was "for the Common Advantage, more especially of the Country Towns."[24] It was specifically aimed at informal practitioners, particularly those in rural areas. In many cases, such practitioners were female. Those who were literate, like Anna Brigham Maynard, could take advantage of the elite knowledge of the author.

Anna Maynard was a member of the Brigham family of Marlborough, Massachusetts, the same family that had preserved the medical wisdom of its women in a notebook for over eighty years. When Maynard asked for and received the smallpox pamphlet, she changed the way medical information entered her family. The pamphlet was written by a stranger, someone known neither to her nor to her kin. It was an impersonal document rather than a personal communication. Like any practitioner, Maynard wanted to have the latest information on the practice of her craft—and in taking advantage of the pamphlet, she added print culture to the oral tradition that had been such an important part of the way the Brigham women practiced healing. By adding the pamphlet to her family's recipes, Maynard also acknowledged the continuing importance of her practice to her patients. She wanted to ensure that the patients who came to her got the best care available.

Thus, Maynard's practice represented a balance between the female traditions and the scientific, regulated future of medicine. Changes in the distribution of information, changes in medical science, the consolidation of the medical profession, and changes in the proper scope of women's work and role within the family came together to change women's medical practice. Anna Maynard recognized this change when she requested the smallpox pamphlet. She felt that information written by a credentialed male expert and dispersed by print was the way of the future, even for lay healers such as herself.

Hannah Parkman and Anna Brigham Maynard were not alone in seeing women's medical practice change around them. While the

Parkmans, the Brighams, and the Maynards were the leading families of a rural, agricultural community, women in other circumstances witnessed the same phenomenon. Mary Viall Holyoke's experience underlines this point. During the latter half of the eighteenth century, in Salem, a sophisticated seaport town, Mary Viall married the physician Edward Augustus Holyoke. Given these circumstances, it might be expected that she would employ male doctors, as indeed she did. Her own husband bled her and lanced her abscessed breast. Seeking a scientific explanation for their many stillborn or short-lived children, Dr. Holyoke performed an autopsy on one of their dead infants in 1770. Mary also trusted herself and her children to her husband's colleagues. In March of 1777, she took her two daughters to a hospital to be inoculated for smallpox and stayed to nurse them through the ordeal. Both girls survived the procedure, although there were some uncertain moments when Judith "had convulsion fits & Betsey Poorly."[25]

Like the Parkman women, Holyoke continued to participate in many of the older social traditions of female medical practice. She had women around her during every medical crisis and for every birth. Some were practitioners; others were her kin and neighbors. Neighbor women watched at the bedside of her dying daughter Polly in 1764, and attended Holyoke's lying-in in 1774. A hired nurse prepared an herbal ointment for Holyoke's sore breast that same month.[26] Female practice did not disappear completely, even in a physician's household.

Mary Holyoke's medical networks also continued to delineate social hierarchies in a town, much as they did in Elizabeth Davenport's time. Her husband Edward was a prominent physician and son of the president of Harvard. As an only child whose parents lived in a distant town, all of Mary's social contacts were with her husband's friends and family. Like Hannah Parkman, Mary was adopted by the family of her husband's first wife, Judith Pickman. Madam Pickman, Judith's mother, attended all of Mary's frequent births and served as a surrogate mother to both Mary and Edward Holyoke.

Like Elizabeth Davenport, Mary Holyoke was a member of a medical network made up of the elite women of her community. Her husband was one of the founding members of the Monday Night Club, a literary and social club.[27] The nonfamily members who visited Mary Holyoke were often the wives, sisters, or daughters of fellow club members—Mrs. Oliver and Mrs. Lynde came during Mary's "sitting up week" in March 1768, and Mary paid similar visits to Mrs. Browne in 1765 and 1769. Edward's medical students contributed other members to Mary's network. Molly Appleton, wife of Nathaniel Appleton, served as nurse to Mary during several of her lying-ins. Once again, the women's medical community followed the same status lines as the larger community.[28]

Despite these continuities, Holyoke's childbed and sickbed visits fit in with a new set of ritualized social calls, especially during the formal sitting up weeks designated for new mothers. Such formal calls reflected the increased gentility and urbanity of some New England communities, especially in important commercial centers like Salem. Formal calls replaced the constant visiting and "gadding" of former times; tea parties replaced communal working parties. Mary Holyoke's luxurious month of sitting up became a part of these calls, with friends arriving to drink tea and chat rather than exchange medical recipes and advice as they would have one hundred years earlier. Nor did Holyoke attend the sick of other social strata; the only mention of this practice was when she paid a visit to a black ex-servant who was dying. Holyoke's postpartum tea parties are a sharp contrast to the functional medical gatherings of Elizabeth Davenport's time.[29]

Indeed, most of the women who came to congratulate Mary on her births did so during her sitting up week, rather than attending the birth itself. When Mary mentioned any activity during that week, it was social, rather than medical, most often drinking tea. Even though women were still gathering at childbeds, the nature of the visits was oriented more toward shared pleasure than shared travail. In Holyoke's diary, visits to the opera and formal balls are recorded in the same entry with visits to women who had just given birth. Women's medical rituals were slowly becoming part of genteel social life, rather than community resources.

In rural areas, women's healing practice lingered longer and remained both more functional and more diverse. As we saw in the case of the Parkmans, women continued to be important members of the medical community even as male doctors moved into the area. One woman, Mrs. Parker, specialized in setting bones and had invested in a complex "apparatus" for her work. Granny Maynard and Anna Brigham Maynard provided important care, especially for women and children. Rural practitioners in general retained more importance. The famous Maine midwife Martha Ballard practiced in the 1810s much as midwives and doctoresses had in the 1630s.[30]

The process of redefining medicine to mean only so-called regular practice (that is, medicine as it was taught in the medical schools of Europe and America) was a long and arduous struggle. Despite physicians' rhetoric condemning "quacks" and "ignorant midwives," in reality they often had no choice but to tolerate and even cooperate with more traditional practitioners. Martha Ballard's early nineteenth-century practice exemplifies this situation. Ballard delivered most of the babies in her Maine town and even attended the wife of the local doctor. Local physicians had great respect for her. They welcomed her presence as a skilled practitioner at the bedsides of women and children; and when Dr. Coleman performed an autopsy on a young boy who had died of burns, he invited Ballard, as a member of the local medical community, to observe.[31]

When a young physician came to the neighborhood, he attempted (as was recommended by many advice books for young doctors) to establish his practice by attending women in labor. The doctor's first attempt was a disaster—the mother and child were only saved by Martha Ballard's timely intervention. However, after Ballard grew too old and frail to continue her practice, her place was taken not by another midwife but by the same doctor whose first attempts at obstetrics had been so clumsy. Even in rural Maine, the paradigm of medical practice had changed by the second decade of the nineteenth century. A medical treatise published shortly after Martha Ballard's death declared that women were too "delicate" to practice midwifery, much less perform surgery or witness dissections. As medicine itself became more concerned with bleeding, dramatic surgical procedures, and violently purgative drugs, it seemed farther and farther removed from the image of women as nurturing, refined, and concerned only with the well-being of their families.[32]

Yet these changes, like others in eighteenth-century medical culture, were uneven and gradual. One example of this phenomenon is the role of female healers in public settings. Despite the professionalization of medicine and the redefinitions of women's role, some aspects of midwifery remained part of the formal public—most saliently, the role of the midwife's testimony in paternity suits and fornication cases. Through the early nineteenth century, midwives continued to make "examinations" of unwed mothers during labor and to testify to the identity of the babies' fathers. Martha Ballard played this role regularly, even when she had to testify that her own son was the father of an illegitimate child.[33]

But even this role was beginning to be redefined as a private rather than a public one. Couples who became pregnant outside of marriage were less and less likely to be prosecuted as criminal fornicators, and men who fathered illegitimate children were less likely to be held criminally responsible. Instead, it was up to the woman and her family to file a civil paternity suit to ensure support for the infant. In this sense, illegitimate babies became a private family problem instead of an offense against the community as a whole. Midwives no longer attended public court days; instead, they gave their testimony in front of a justice of the peace. The criminal and high-level civil courts were redefined as purely male territory. As a result, the social authority of the midwife as a representative of community values was diminished. Women's sexuality, reproduction, and medical problems became part of a restricted private sphere, and women practitioners, such as midwives, also were relegated to that sphere.[34]

As medical schools and professional physicians proliferated in the first half of the nineteenth century, there were new calls for educated female doctors and a public role for female healers from diverse segments of society. From social conservatives concerned about women's modesty, to women's rights activists concerned with women's opportunities, advocates for women's practice used the new construction of womanhood to argue in favor women's practice. Since women were by nature gentle, nurturing, and caring, they should make excellent doctors, and since women were also by nature modest and shy, they should have female caretakers to shield them from the prying eyes and hands of men. Underlying these arguments, particularly those of the feminists, was the assumption that women could and should have a role to play in the redefined public world. Having women enter the medical profession would be one step toward having them enter the "formal public" that had been redefined as exclusively male.

If Martha Ballard was a transitional figure with her roots in the colonial period, Harriot K. Hunt of Boston pointed toward the scientific and social concerns of the nineteenth century. Hunt was born in 1805, seven years before Martha Ballard died. Like many of her colonial forebears, Hunt learned her craft from another woman in an informal apprenticeship. She met her preceptor, Mrs. Mott, in 1833 when Hunt's sister was incapacitated by illness. Mrs. Mott effected a successful cure. Afterward, both Hunt and her sister were inspired to take up the practice of medicine themselves. Mrs. Mott educated the Hunts in her own blend of herbal medicine, hydropathy, phrenology, and hygiene. Hunt supplemented her apprenticeship with extensive independent reading, as did literate colonial women and most colonial physicians. She practiced for forty years, tending mostly to women and children.[35]

Despite this old-style education and practice, Harriot Hunt was not conscious of the tradition in which she was participating. Instead, she looked steadfastly into the future. In her memoir, *Glances and Glimpses*, she emphasized over and over the scientific basis of her cures, and optimistically looked forward to future advances in both medicine and other technology. Underlying this attitude toward science and medicine was Hunt's intense desire to enter the professional practice of medicine on the same basis as men. Indeed, the biggest disappointment of her life, and the incident for which she is best known today, is her failure to be admitted to Harvard Medical College. She applied twice—once, in 1847, when the faculty rejected her application, and once more in 1850, when she convinced the faculty to admit her, but the student body successfully petitioned for her rejection. Hunt deeply regretted the gaps in her education: "General and special anatomy—shall I ever forgive the Harvard Medical College for depriving me of a thorough knowledge of that science?"[36] Unlike her seventeenth- and eighteenth-century forebears, Hunt located medical practice exclusively in the public sphere. Without a man's education and professional credentials, she felt that her practice could never be legitimate. Instead of working cooperatively with male physicians in a hierarchical relationship, Hunt wanted to hang out a shingle and compete directly with other practitioners on an equal basis.

This desire for women's participation in the public world of commerce and politics also manifests itself in the links Hunt saw between women's medical practice and the social and political issues of the day. She thought medicine was essential to the cure of the many social ills she saw around her. She felt that physicians—not just any physicians, but properly educated female physicians—had a special role to play

in solving these problems. In her memoir, Hunt wrote on issues ranging from the suffering of poor widows, to the sexual exploitation of
young girls, to the problems created by drunkenness—all of which she
connected to health issues and her own medical practice.

For instance, Hunt described the "heart history" of a sixteen-year-
old girl who came to Boston thinking to marry a wealthy man. Instead of marrying her, her "fiancé" seduced and abandoned her. The
experience had an effect on the girl's physical health: "A leaden dull-
ness seized this beautiful child; the ruddy glow vanished from her
face; symmetry of form was gone; a pallid languor overspread her
features; mind and soul were blighted; and a feeling of repulsion,
blended with tenderness for the fallen, filled my mind."[37] Hunt linked
this phenomenon with the increasing disparity between rich and poor
in the rapidly growing city: "Profligacy is very general, and is shame-
fully tolerated; houses of assignation abound; their bolted doors
swing open noiselessly to the clink of a heavy purse."[38] Similarly,
Hunt took up the cause of temperance. She attributed her interest in
the issue to having seen a "beautiful woman" afflicted with delirium
tremens: "It was a fearful shock to my nervous system. Disheveled
hair, glaring eyes, partial nudity, in one of my own sex, was terrific to
me." Her experience brought home the "sins and the wretchedness
that grow out of this everyday vice."[39]

Hunt linked these sociomedical problems with the oppression of
women, especially poor women. She noted that she had been "for fif-
teen years the confidant of woman, who had known that her diseases
resulted in great measure from her position; who had sympathized
with the heart-broken, prescribed for the penniless, and mingled her
tears with the widow and the fatherless."[40]

With these issues in mind, Hunt became a supporter of the early
women's movement. She not only wanted better conditions for her
patients but also wanted recognition and approval for women physicians like herself. She called the movement "bread and water to my
soul."[41] Hunt described in great detail her attendance at the first national women's rights convention in Worcester, Massachusetts, in
1850. She wrote with particular approval of Sarah Tyndale, who when
"left a widow with a family of children dependent on her exertions,
she continued her husband's business." Tyndale spoke in the hope
that "she might encourage every widow and raise her voice against
the narrow sphere prescribed to woman."[42] In this, Hunt and Tyndale

were alike. Both wanted women to enter the public sphere on the same basis as men. Hunt saw medicine, work, feminism, politics, and women's health as parts of a whole. All these issues, and the host of social ills she connected with them, could be addressed by allowing women to practice medicine as credentialed professionals.

Elizabeth Blackwell was the woman who would succeed in bringing these aspirations to fruition. When she entered Geneva Medical College in 1847 on her way to becoming the first regular woman physician in the United States, her choice was based on both women's rights concerns and a conventional view of nineteenth-century womanhood. Blackwell grew up in a remarkable family of social and moral reformers. Her father was an antislavery activist; her sister Emily would follow her into the practice of medicine; her brothers continued their father's activism. Blackwell's brothers demonstrated their commitment to women's rights by marrying feminist women. Henry Blackwell married suffragist Lucy Stone, and Samuel married Antoinette Brown, the first ordained woman minister in the nation. Given this family background, it is not surprising that Blackwell chose an unconventional life and dedicated herself to reform principles.[43]

Like Harriot Hunt and her other peers in the temperance, moral reform, and alternative-health movements, Blackwell assumed that women had special traits. Most notable of these traits were an innate moral intuition and an instinct for nurturing and healing, all of which stemmed from the female capacity for motherhood. Blackwell cited these traits as one of her motivations for the study of medicine, writing in her memoir, "I have always felt a great reverence for maternity—the mighty creative power which more than any other human faculty seemed to bring womanhood nearer the Divine."[44] This power may have originated with motherhood, but Blackwell also saw it as necessary to the practice of medicine.

Blackwell shared with Hunt the assumption that these traits, originally designed to help women make homes and raise children, had a place in the public world. Indeed, Blackwell saw women physicians not only as necessary to their patients but also as crucial elements in the moral progress of the United States as a whole: "We may look forward with hope to the future influence of Christian women physicians, when with sympathy and reverence guiding intellectual activity they learn to apply the vital principles of their Great Master to every method and practice of the healing art." Blackwell chose medicine, despite her personal distaste for "the physical," because of this strong "moral element."[45] While this model of both womanhood and medicine would soon be under attack by other women doctors, it was the model that originally attracted women like Blackwell to the field.[46]

With Blackwell's entrance into medical school, women's medical practice had come full circle: from work that women did within a "women's public" and that brought some female practitioners into the male public of the courts, to a purely private act women performed in the service of their families, to a public practice once again, performed in the service of the nation. Elizabeth Blackwell thought of herself as a trailblazer for women doctors and for women patients, as the title of her memoir, *Pioneer Work in Opening the Medical Profession to Women*, demonstrates. What she and her readers may not have been aware of, however, was that she was not the first woman healer in America. Elizabeth Blackwell was only one link in the long chain of women's practice.

Notes

Preface

1. Entries for January 2–16, 1702, in M. Halsey Thomas, ed., *The Diary of Samuel Sewall*, vol. 1 (New York: Farrar, Straus and Giroux, 1973), pp. 459–60.

2. 30-18-3, Essex County Court File Papers, Essex Institute, Salem, Mass. (microfilm, Yale University, New Haven, Conn.).

3. This description of the calling is based on Edmund Morgan's in *The Puritan Family: Religion and Domestic Relations in Seventeenth-Century New England* (New York: Harper and Row, 1944), pp. 66–78.

Chapter 1. CALLING THE HEALERS

1. Charles Brigham Account Book, 1650–1730, Folder Five, American Antiquarian Society, Worcester, Mass.

2. For a thorough discussion of this issue in seventeenth-century England, see Lucinda McCray Beier, *Sufferers and Healers: The Experience of Illness in Seventeenth-Century England* (London: Routledge and Kegan Paul, 1987).

3. George E. Gifford, "Botanic Remedies in Colonial Massachusetts, 1620–1820," in J. Worth Estes, ed., *Medicine in Colonial Massachusetts, 1620–1820* (Boston: Colonial Society of Massachusetts, 1978), pp. 263–88; Edward Eggleston, *The Transit of Civilization from England to America in the Seventeenth Century* (New York: Appleton, 1901), pp. 48–95; Lester S. King, "The Transformation of Galenism," in Alan G. Debus, ed., *Medicine in Seventeenth-Century England* (Berkeley: University of California Press, 1974), pp. 7–32.

4. Eggleston, *Transit of Civilization*, p. 62.

5. Thomas Palmer, *The Admirable Secrets of Physick and Chyrurgery*, ed. Thomas Rogers Forbes (New Haven: Yale University Press, 1984), p. 2.

6. Cotton Mather, *The Angel of Bethesda: An Essay upon the Common Maladies of Mankind*, ed. Gordon W. Jones (Barre, Mass.: American Antiquarian Society and Barre Publishers, 1972), p. xxii.

7. Nancy G. Siraisi, *Medieval and Early Renaissance Medicine: An Introduction to Knowledge and Practice* (Chicago: University of Chicago Press, 1990), p. 117; see also Alfred White Franklin, "Clinical Medicine," in Debus, ed., *Medicine in Seventeenth-Century England*, pp. 113–45.

8. Nicholas Culpeper, *Pharmacopoeia Londoniensis: or the London Dispensatory further adorned by the studies and collections of the fellows now living, of the said college* (Boston: Printed by John Allen for Nicholas Boone at the Sign of the Bible in Cornhill, 1720), p. 272. Culpeper's original herbal was published in London in 1652.

9. Gifford, "Botanic Remedies," pp. 263–65.

10. Ibid., p. 264; Mather, *Angel of Bethesda*, p. xxiii; Charles Webster, *The Great Instauration: Science, Medicine, and Reform, 1626–1660* (London: Duckworth, 1975).

11. Gifford, "Botanic Remedies," esp. p. 264.

12. Beier, *Sufferers and Healers*, pp. 168–70. This mentality persisted into nineteenth-century practice; see John Harley Warner, *The Therapeutic Perspective: Medical Practice, Knowledge, and Identity in America, 1820–1885* (Cambridge: Harvard University Press, 1986).

13. John Davenport to John Winthrop Jr., December 17, 1660, in Isabel MacBeath Calder, ed., *The Letters of John Davenport, Puritan Divine* (New Haven: Yale University Press, 1937), p. 185.

14. Doreen Evenden Nagy, *Popular Medicine in Seventeenth-Century England* (Bowling Green, Ohio: Bowling Green University Popular Press, 1988), p. 53.

15. Beier, *Sufferers and Healers*, pp. 173–81.

16. Nagy, *Popular Medicine*, pp. 5–7.

17. Charles Brigham Account Book, Folder Five.

18. Palmer, *Admirable Secrets of Physick and Chyrurgery*, p. 130.

19. Siraisi, *Medieval and Early Renaissance Medicine*, p. 140. Whitfield Bell notes that in Philadelphia some practitioners offered bleeding as a specialized practice like midwifery or bonesetting. Whitfield J. Bell Jr., "Medicine in Boston and Philadelphia: Comparisons and Contrasts, 1750–1820," in Estes, ed., *Medicine in Colonial Massachusetts*, pp. 159–81; 32-21-1, Essex County Court File Papers, Essex Institute, Salem, Mass. (microfilm, Yale University, New Haven, Conn.); Palmer, *Admirable Secrets of Physick and Chyrurgery*, pp. 49–50.

20. Diary of Ebenezer Parkman, 1756–1761, Parkman Family Papers, American Antiquarian Society, Worcester, Mass.

21. My thanks to Professor Ross Beales of the College of the Holy Cross for running the computer search that turned up this statistic. Even though only men performed bleedings, a few women kept notes or charts indicating the most propitious times for bleeding. For an example of such a chart, see Dorothy Cotton's notes on the influence of the moon on such things as childbirth, sickness, and bleeding that she wrote in her husband Seaborn's journal. This document is reproduced as "The Nature and Disposition of the Moon in the Birth of Children," in John Demos, ed., *Remarkable Providences: Readings on Early American History* (Boston: Northeastern University Press, 1991), pp. 440–46. Even though Dorothy Cotton kept track of the best days to draw blood, there is no evidence that she drew the blood herself.

22. Siraisi, *Medieval and Early Renaissance Medicine*, p. 141; William C. Wigglesworth, "Surgery in Massachusetts, 1620–1800," in Estes, ed., *Medicine in Colonial Massachusetts*, pp. 227–48.

23. William Leete to John Winthrop Jr., March 29, 1658; William Leete to John Winthrop Jr., June 22, 1658, in *The Winthrop Papers*, Collections of the Massachusetts Historical Society, 4th series, vol. 7 (Boston: Massachusetts Historical Society, 1865), pp. 539–41.

24. David Hackett Fischer, *Albion's Seed: Four British Folkways in America* (New York: Oxford University Press, 1989), p. 132. See also David D. Hall, *Worlds of Won-*

der, *Days of Judgment: Popular Religious Belief in Early New England* (Cambridge: Harvard University Press, 1989), pp. 21–70.

25. Rhys Isaac, "Books and the Social Authority of Learning: The Case of Mid-Eighteenth-Century Virginia," in William L. Joyce et al., eds., *Printing and Society in Early America* (Worcester, Mass.: American Antiquarian Society, 1983), pp. 228–49, quotation on p. 239.

26. Mather, *Angel of Bethesda*, p. xxxiii.

27. John Barton Account Book, 1662–1676, American Antiquarian Society, Worcester, Mass.

28. Dressing servant's leg, 22-82-1, Essex County Court File Papers; mention in probate inventory, Inventory of Richard Langhorne, *Records and Files of the Quarterly Courts of Essex County*, vol. 5 (Salem: Essex Institute, 1911), p. 442.

29. Mary Beth Norton, *Founding Mothers and Fathers: Gendered Power and the Forming of American Society* (New York: Knopf, 1996), p. 362.

30. W. I. Tyler Brigham, *The History of the Brigham Family*, vol. 1 (New York: Grafton Press, 1907), pp. 116–17; entries for November 1759 and October 1758, in Diary of Ebenezer Parkman, Parkman Family Papers.

31. Entries for July 9 and 10, 1759, in Diary of Ebenezer Parkman, Parkman Family Papers.

32. Charles Brigham Account Book, Folders Three and Four.

33. Palmer, *Admirable Secrets of Physick and Chyrurgery*, pp. 24–25.

34. Ibid., p. 23.

35. Ibid., p. 34.

36. C. Helen Brock, "The Influence of Europe on Colonial Massachusetts Medicine," in Estes, ed., *Medicine in Colonial Massachusetts*, pp. 101–44.

37. William Eamon, *Science and the Secrets of Nature: Books of Secrets in Medieval and Early Modern Culture* (Princeton: Princeton University Press, 1994).

38. Ibid., p. 356.

39. Ibid., pp. 134–67.

40. Michael Warner, "The Public Sphere and the Cultural Mediation of Print," in William S. Solomon and Robert W. McChesney, eds., *Ruthless Criticism: New Perspectives in U.S. Communications History* (Minneapolis: University of Minnesota Press, 1993), pp. 7–37, quotation on p. 21.

41. Ibid.; Jill Lepore, *The Name of War: King Philip's War and the Origin of American Identity* (New York: Knopf, 1998), pp. 21–47; Hall, *Worlds of Wonder, Days of Judgment*, pp. 21–70.

42. Warner, "The Public Sphere and the Cultural Mediation of Print," pp. 20–22.

43. Tamara Plakins Thornton, *Handwriting in America: A Cultural History* (New Haven: Yale University Press, 1996), p. 23.

44. Ibid., pp. 22–24.

Chapter 2. CALLED TO THE BEDSIDE

1. This description of a sickbed scene is based on a recipe for sack posset and suggestions for its use found in the Charles Brigham Account Book, 1650–1730, Folder One, American Antiquarian Society, Worcester, Mass.

2. W. I. Tyler Brigham, *The History of the Brigham Family: A Record of Several Thousand Descendants of Thomas Brigham the Emigrant, 1603–1653* (New York: Grafton Press, 1907), 2 vols.

3. Charles Brigham Account Book, Folder One, Folder Two.

4. *A Book of Fruits and Flowers* (Exeter, England: Rota, 1978), p. 17.

5. Charles Brigham Account Book, Folder One (fricassee of chickens), Folder Four (plague), Folder Six (medlar preserves).

6. Nancy G. Siraisi, *Medieval and Early Renaissance Medicine: An Introduction to Knowledge and Practice* (Chicago: University of Chicago Press, 1990), p. 121.

7. Gervase Markham, *The English Housewife* (London: Nicholas Oakes, 1631), p. 4.

8. John Josselyn, "New England's Rarities Discovered," *Transactions and Collections of the American Antiquarian Society*, vol. 4 (1860; reprint, 1971), pp. 220–24.

9. John Davenport to John Winthrop Jr., December 23, 1660, in Isabel MacBeath Calder, ed., *The Letters of John Davenport, Puritan Divine* (New Haven: Yale University Press, 1937), pp. 186–87.

10. Markham, *English Housewife*, p. 149.

11. Daniel Leeds, *An Almanac and Ephemerides for the Year of Christian Account 1693, by Daniel Leeds, Philomath* ([Boston?]: William Bradford, 1693), end pages.

12. John Evelyn, *Kalendrium Hortense: or, the Gard'ners Almanac* (London, 1666), p. 52; John B. Lust, *The Herb Book* (New York: Bantam, 1974), p. 179.

13. Charles Brigham Account Book, Folder One.

14. The earliest reference to a stilled medicine in America dates from 1666. From the correspondence between John Davenport and John Winthrop Jr.: "Mrs. Bache her water made of mint and sack and saunders distilled." John Davenport to John Winthrop Jr., May 1, 1666, in Calder, ed., *Letters of John Davenport*, p. 261. While this was the earliest reference I could find to a stilled medicine, stilling was probably in use from the time of the first European settlements.

15. Recipe for "The Greater Palsie Water," in Charles Brigham Account Book, Folder Two.

16. Charles Brigham Account Book, Folder Three.

17. John Davenport to John Winthrop Jr., September 17, 1654, in Calder, ed., *Letters of John Davenport*, p. 97.

18. Testimony of Hannah Hazen, Mary Leaver, and Mary Leighton, 37-73-4, Essex County Court File Papers, Essex Institute, Salem, Mass. (microfilm, Yale University, New Haven, Conn.).

19. Lucinda McCray Beier, *Sufferers and Healers: The Experience of Illness in Seventeenth-Century England* (London: Routledge and Kegan Paul, 1987), pp. 40–41; see also Wyndam B. Blanton, *Medicine in Virginia in the Seventeenth Century* (Richmond: William Byrd, 1930), pp. 141–44; Thomas Palmer, *The Admirable Secrets of Physick and Chyrurgery*, ed. Thomas Rogers Forbes (New Haven: Yale University Press, 1984), pp. 41–42; and Siraisi, *Medieval and Early Renaissance Medicine*, pp. 124–25. Siraisi notes that medieval practitioners made similar diagnoses using blood—letting it stand and noting its "viscosity, hotness . . . coldness, 'greasiness,' taste, foaminess, rapidity of coagulation, and the characteristics of the layers into which drawn blood separated" (p. 124). This practice was never as widespread as uroscopy, and seems to have disappeared completely by the seventeenth century. "Piss prophet" quotation in Cotton Mather, *The Angel of Bethesda: An Essay upon the Common Maladies of Mankind*, ed. Gordon W. Jones (Barre, Mass.: American Antiquarian Society and Barre Publishers, 1972), p. 251.

20. John Davenport to John Winthrop Jr., July 20, 1660, December 17, 1660, and December 23, 1660, in Calder, ed., *Letters of John Davenport*, pp. 167, 185, 188.

21. Dr. John Barton of Salem, Massachusetts, noted that if blood formed a black sediment in the urine flask, it indicated a bladder stone; orange-colored urine in-

dicated inflammation of the liver. John Barton Account Book, American Antiquarian Society, Worcester, Mass.

22. For examples of these practices, see entries for January 9, 1739, in Francis G. Walett, ed., *The Diary of Ebenezer Parkman, 1703–1782* (Worcester, Mass.: American Antiquarian Society, 1974), p. 59; also entries for month of April 1759 in Diary of Ebenezer Parkman, 1756–1761, Parkman Family Papers, American Antiquarian Society, Worcester, Mass.; and entries for the month of January 1764 in "Diary of Mary Viall Holyoke," in George Francis Dow, ed., *The Holyoke Diaries* (Salem: Essex Institute, 1911).

23. Entry for May 16, 1709, in Worthington Chauncy Ford, ed., *The Diary of Cotton Mather*, vol. 2 (New York: Frederick Ungar, 1957), pp. 8–9; entry for November 30, 1750, in Walett, ed., *Diary of Ebenezer Parkman*, p. 228.

24. 22-83-1, Essex County Court File Papers. The entire case is contained in files 22-80-1, 82-1, 83-1, 83-3, 83-4, 84-1.

25. John Pynchon to John Winthrop Jr., May 28, 1655, in Carl Bridenbaugh, ed., *The Pynchon Papers*, vol. 1 (Boston: Colonial Society of Massachusetts, 1982), pp. 14–16; John Pynchon to John Winthrop Jr., May 28, 1655, in ibid.; entry for October 25, 1725, in Walett, ed., *Diary of Ebenezer Parkman*, p. 7.

26. Charles Brigham Account Book, Folder Four.

27. The following description of a "typical" illness is a composite based on the following sources: Charles Brigham Account Book, especially the directions in Folder Four for nursing a person through the plague; Cotton Mather, *A Letter, about a good management under the distemper of the measles at this time spreading in the country* (Boston: Printed and Sold by Thomas Fleet at the Heart and Crown in Cornhill, 1739); Thomas Thacher, *A brief rule to guide the common people of New-England: how to order themselves and theirs in the small pox, or measels* (Boston: Printed and sold by John Foster, 1677); and from the various sources cited above.

28. "Directions for prevention in the time of the Plague or Pestilence," Charles Brigham Account Book, Folder Four.

29. Mather, *A Letter*, p. 3.

30. Like the description of illness, this description of a "typical" childbirth is a composite, based primarily on two midwifery manuals: Jane Sharp, *The Midwives Book* (1671; reprint, New York: Garland, 1985); *Aristotle's Compleat Masterpiece: In Three Parts: Displaying the secrets of nature in the generation of man. Regularly digested in chapters and sections, rendering it far more useful and easy than any yet extant*, 26th ed. ([London?]: Printed and Sold by the booksellers, 1755); and numerous descriptions of travails in court records, letters, and diaries cited throughout.

31. John B. D'Emilio and Estelle B. Freedman, *Intimate Matters: A History of Sexuality in America* (New York: Harper and Row, 1988), pp. 16–27; Catherine Scholten, *Childbearing in American Society, 1650–1850* (New York: New York University Press, 1985), pp. 13–14; Susan E. Klepp, "Lost, Hidden, Obstructed, and Repressed: Contraceptive and Abortive Technology in the Early Delaware Valley," in Judith A. McGaw, ed., *Early American Technology: Making and Doing Things from the Colonial Era to 1850* (Chapel Hill: University of North Carolina Press, 1994), pp. 68–113; Cornelia Hughes Dayton, "Taking the Trade: Abortion and Gender Relations in an Eighteenth-Century New England Village," *William and Mary Quarterly*, 3rd series, 158 (1991): 19–49.

32. Charles Brigham Account Book, Folder Five.

33. Lust, *Herb Book*. Styptic and astringent herbs in this recipe include plantain, sanicle, oak leaves, dandelion, water avens, blackberry or bramble buds, cinquefoil, and betony.

34. Charles Brigham Account Book, Folder Four.

35. Lust, *Herb Book*, pp. 243, 260, 282, 284, 341, 379. Savin seems to have been the most common early American abortifacient. See Dayton, "Taking the Trade"; and Julia Cherry Spruill, *Women's Life and Work in the Southern Colonies* (1938; reprint, New York: Norton, 1972), pp. 325–27. Klepp, in "Lost, Hidden, Obstructed, and Repressed," discusses a wide range of abortifacient herbs and techniques, including juniper berries, madder roots, and snakeroot—another name for the "sanicle" mentioned in the Brighams' recipe.

36. Klepp, "Lost, Hidden, Obstructed, and Repressed," pp. 76–81.

37. *Aristotle's Compleat Masterpiece*, pp. 39–40.

38. Klepp, "Lost, Hidden, Obstructed and Repressed," p. 73.

39. Case of Hannah Blood, 1677-79-2, Middlesex County Court File Papers, Massachusetts Archives, Columbia Point, Boston.

40. Dayton, "Taking the Trade," p. 23; discussion of early American prosecutions for abortion, p. 20.

41. David D. Hall, *Worlds of Wonder, Days of Judgment: Popular Religious Belief in Early New England* (Cambridge: Harvard University Press, 1989), pp. 196–210.

42. Richard Godbeer, *The Devil's Dominion: Magic and Religion in Early New England* (New York: Cambridge University Press, 1992), p. 16. See also Jon Butler, *Awash in a Sea of Faith: Christianizing the American People* (Cambridge: Harvard University Press, 1990), pp. 67–97; and on folk magic in English society, see Keith Thomas, *Religion and the Decline of Magic* (New York: Scribner's, 1971).

43. Talman Family Papers, Series 1, General Documents, Folder Four, Manuscripts and Archives, Yale University, New Haven, Conn.

44. John Barton Account Book.

45. Thomas, *Religion and the Decline of Magic*, p. 191. Thomas includes a lengthy discussion of magical cures, pp. 177–211.

46. Entry for October 22, 1702, in Ford, ed., *Diary of Cotton Mather*, vol. 1., p. 444.

47. For more on the uneasy coexistence of magic and religion in New England, see Godbeer, *Devil's Dominion*.

48. Entry for April 2, 1677, in M. Halsey Thomas, ed., *The Diary of Samuel Sewall*, vol. 1 (New York: Farrar, Straus and Giroux, 1973), p. 41.

49. Charles Brigham Account Book, Folder Three.

50. Thomas, *Religion and the Decline of Magic*, p. 624.

51. Charles Brigham Account Book, Folder Four.

52. Thomas, *Religion and the Decline of Magic*, pp. 183–86, esp. p. 184.

53. Charles Brigham Account Book, Folder Three.

54. Astrological medicine was an area where magic and science were not entirely distinguished. For one thing, astrology and astronomy were still closely related; for another, people of the time saw sound reasons to believe that the stars had a natural influence on earthly events. Like Kenelm Digby's wound salve, astrological medicine was an area where some practitioners thought of themselves as effecting natural cures; others, supernatural ones. Nor was astrology incompatible with Christian piety. For a detailed discussion of early modern astrology and its relationship to medicine, science, and religion, see Thomas, *Religion and*

the Decline of Magic, pp. 283–385; and Butler, *Awash in a Sea of Faith,* pp. 20–25; and for the relationship between medical science and medical astrology, see Siraisi, *Medieval and Early Renaissance Medicine,* pp. 135–36. Michael MacDonald's *Mystical Bedlam: Madness, Anxiety, and Healing in Seventeenth-Century England* (New York: Cambridge University Press, 1981) gives an in-depth description of the practice of Richard Napier, a well-known astrological physician.

55. Testimony of Mary Godfrey, in Nathaniel Bouton, ed., *Documents and Records Relating to the Province of New Hampshire,* vol. 1 (Concord, N.H.: George E. Jenks, State Printer, 1867), p. 416.

56. Testimony of Mary Godfrey and testimony of Nathaniel Smith, in ibid., pp. 416, 417–18. John Putnam Demos includes a discussion of this case in *Entertaining Satan: Witchcraft and the Culture of New England* (New York: Oxford University Press, 1982), pp. 330–32.

57. Barbara Ehrenreich and Deirdre English, *Witches, Midwives and Nurses: A History of Women Healers* (Old Westbury, N.Y.: Feminist Press, 1973). Ehrenreich and English are not professional historians, and their agenda in writing this book was not a scholarly one. However, their argument that women healers were particularly vulnerable to witchcraft accusations has found its way into scholarly treatments of witchcraft as well. Both John Demos *(Entertaining Satan)* and Carol Karlsen (cited below) devote portions of their work to addressing this issue.

58. Alan MacFarlane, *Witchcraft in Tudor and Stuart England: A Regional and Comparative Study* (Prospect Heights, Ill.: Waveland Press, 1970), pp. 152–53; Carol Karlsen, *The Devil in the Shape of a Woman: Witchcraft in Colonial New England* (New York: Norton, 1987), pp. 145–46.

Chapter 3. CALLING THE WOMEN

1. Entries for December 26–28, 1738, in Francis G. Walett, ed., *The Diary of Ebenezer Parkman, 1703–1782* (Worcester, Mass.: American Antiquarian Society, 1974), p. 56.

2. Mary Beth Norton, *Founding Mothers and Fathers: Gendered Power and the Forming of American Society* (New York: Knopf, 1996), p. 19.

3. Judith Walzer Leavitt, *Brought to Bed: Childbearing in America, 1750–1950* (New York: Oxford University Press, 1986), pp. 87–115.

4. Entries for August 12–13, 1690, in M. Halsey Thomas, ed., *The Diary of Samuel Sewall,* vol. 1 (New York: Farrar, Straus and Giroux, 1973), p. 264.

5. Entry for May 16, 1709, in Worthington Chauncey Ford, ed., *Diary of Cotton Mather,* vol. 2 (New York: Frederick Ungar, 1957), pp. 8–9.

6. *Aristotle's Compleat Masterpiece: In Three Parts: Displaying the secrets of nature in the generation of man. Regularly digested in chapters and sections, rendering it far more useful and easy than any yet extant,* 26th ed. ([London?]: Printed and Sold by the booksellers, 1755), pp. 66, 69.

7. Entry for February 18, 1747, in Walett, ed., *Diary of Ebenezer Parkman,* p. 150.

8. Entries for November 21, 1694, and January 16, 1702, in Thomas, ed., *Diary of Samuel Sewall,* vol. 1, pp. 324, 459–60.

9. "Diary of Mary Viall Holyoke," in George Francis Dow, ed., *The Holyoke Diaries* (Salem: Essex Institute, 1911). See, for example, the entries for February 14–17, 1773, on p. 82.

10. *Records of the Suffolk County Court, 1671–1680*, Publications of the Colonial Society of Massachusetts, vol. 30 (Boston: Colonial Society of Massachusetts, 1933), p. 839.

11. 45-122-1, Essex County Court File Papers, Essex Institute, Salem, Mass. (microfilm, Yale University, New Haven, Conn.).

12. John Davenport to John Winthrop Jr., May 1, 1666, in Isabel MacBeath Calder, ed., *The Letters of John Davenport, Puritan Divine* (New Haven: Yale University Press, 1937), p. 261; John Davenport to John Winthrop, May 1, 1666, in ibid., pp. 261–62.

13. William Leete to John Winthrop Jr., March 29, 1658, in *The Winthrop Papers*, Collections of the Massachusetts Historical Society, 4th series, vol. 7 (Boston: Massachusetts Historical Society, 1865), p. 539.

14. Entries for February 7–8, 1739, in Walett, ed., *Diary of Ebenezer Parkman*, p. 60.

15. Cotton Mather, *The Angel of Bethesda: An Essay upon the Common Maladies of Mankind*, ed. Gordon W. Jones (Barre: American Antiquarian Society and Barre Publishers, 1972), p. 237.

16. Norton, *Founding Mothers and Fathers*, p. 222.

17. Charles E. Hambrick-Stowe, *The Practice of Piety: Puritan Devotional Disciplines in Seventeenth-Century New England* (Chapel Hill: University of North Carolina Press, 1982), pp. 140–41.

18. Daniel Scott Smith, "'All in Some Degree Related to Each Other': A Demographic and Comparative Resolution of the Anomaly of New England Kinship," *American Historical Review* 94 (1989): 44–79, quotation on 73; Helena M. Wall, *Fierce Communion: Family and Community in Early America* (Cambridge: Harvard University Press, 1990).

19. David Cressy, *Coming Over: Migration and Communication between England and New England in the Seventeenth Century* (New York: Cambridge University Press, 1987), pp. 275–78, quotation on p. 275; David Cressy, "Kinship and Kin Interaction in Early Modern England," *Past and Present* 113 (1986): 38–69, quotation on 51.

20. Marriage to Hannah Breck, footnote to entry for September 24, 1737; miscarriage, entries for February 20–28, 1738, in Walett, ed., *Diary of Ebenezer Parkman*, pp. 41, 45.

21. Ruth Hicks, entry for January 5, 1739; "lower limbs grow useless," entry for January 19, 1739; Elizabeth Champney Winchester, entry for January 21, 1739; measles, entry for March 27, 1740; Ebenezer's illness, entries for November 17 and 22, 1739; Hannah's fall, entry for December 2, 1739; all in ibid., pp. 59, 76, 71.

22. Entries for August 20, 1727, February 20, 1738, December 25, 1739, March 13, 1745, February 1747, January 27, 1749, August 22, 1751, October 18, 1755, in ibid., pp. 27, 45, 56, 72, 113, 150, 190, 242, 296.

23. Entries for January 17, 1726 (Molly's illness), December 26, 1739 (the grave), January 12–13, 1746 (Hannah's illness), in ibid., pp. 15, 72, 130.

24. Entries for December 28, 1738 (Hannah's childbed), November 30, 1750 (Billy cuts his foot), August 24–26, 1752 (Ebenezer's illness), in ibid., pp. 56, 228, 250.

25. Entries for January 22, 1757 (Hepzibah comes to dine), and October 23, 1757 (funeral), in Diary of Ebenezer Parkman, 1756–1761, Parkman Family Papers, American Antiquarian Society, Worcester, Mass.

26. *Westborough Vital Records* (Worcester, Mass.: Franklin P. Rice, 1903), p. 128.

27. For examples of visits, see entries for April 30, 1750, November 23, 1752, and February 24, 1745; "excellent flax seed," entry for April 6, 1747, in Walett, ed., *Diary of Ebenezer Parkman*, pp. 215, 264, 112, 152.

28. Gifts from the Maynards, entry for January 7, 1756; gift to Mary, March 22, 1758; in Diary of Ebenezer Parkman, Parkman Family Papers.

29. For a detailed discussion of the "women's economy" and its connection to women's medical practice, see Laurel Thatcher Ulrich, *A Midwife's Tale: The Life of Martha Ballard Based on Her Diary, 1785–1812* (New York: Knopf, 1990), pp. 72–101. Networks of adopted kin that depend on elaborate barter exchanges for survival are not unknown in the twentieth century. Among impoverished inner-city residents, such networks are common. Anthropologist Carol Stack argues that this strategy makes sense under circumstances when goods and cash are scarce—a situation that describes seventeenth- and eighteenth-century Massachusetts as well as twentieth-century midwestern cities. See Carol B. Stack, *All Our Kin: Strategies for Survival in a Black Community* (New York: Harper and Row, 1974).

30. Norton, *Founding Mothers and Fathers*, p. 248.

31. John Putnam Demos, *Entertaining Satan: Witchcraft and the Culture of Early New England* (New York: Oxford University Press, 1982), pp. 347–48.

32. "The Kellys describe their daughter's fatal illness" in David D. Hall, ed., *Witch-Hunting in Seventeenth-Century New England: A Documentary History* (Boston: Northeastern University Press, 1991), p. 152.

33. Ibid., p. 153.

34. Ibid.

35. Ibid.

36. "Witnesses to the Appearance of the Kellys' child," "An Autopsy Report on John Kelly's Child," and "John Whiting describes the 'possesssion' of Ann Cole," in Hall, ed., *Witch-Hunting*, pp. 154–55, 148–51.

37. For other discussions of Harrison's case, see Richard Godbeer, *The Devil's Dominion: Magic and Religion in Early New England* (New York: Cambridge University Press, 1992), pp. 33–34; and Carol F. Karlsen, *The Devil in the Shape of a Woman: Witchcraft in Colonial New England* (New York: Norton, 1997), pp. 84–89.

38. Demos, *Entertaining Satan*, p. 352; "Hanna Robbins reports her father's suspicions" in Hall, ed., *Witch-Hunting*, p. 157.

39. "Alice Wakely on Mrs. Robbins Body," in Hall, ed., *Witch-Hunting*, pp. 157–58. The consequences for Harrison did not come to fruition for another six years. She escaped trial during the Hartford witch-hunt; instead, the accusation made in 1662 meant years and years of suspicions, accusations, and finally, a trial for witchcraft in 1668. In her final trial, other women's testimonies concerning Harrison's medical practice figured prominently. The jury could not reach a verdict, and the presiding magistrates ordered her to leave the colony. Harrison moved to New York, where she was once again accused of witchcraft in 1670.

40. "Joseph Marsh testifies against Goodwife Ayres," in Hall, ed., *Witch-Hunting*, pp. 155–56.

41. "John Whiting describes the 'possession' of Ann Cole," in ibid., pp. 148–50.

42. "The Swimming Test" and "The Greensmiths are Indicted; the jury convicts them," in ibid., pp. 151–52.

43. Introduction to the Hartford Witch Hunt, in ibid., pp. 147–48.

44. On kin relations, see Wall, *Fierce Communion*; and John Demos, *A Little Commonwealth: Family Life in Plymouth Colony* (New York: Oxford University Press, 1990); on the role of business in creating communities, see Stephen Innes, *To Labor in a New Land: Economy and Society in Seventeenth-Century Springfield* (Princeton:

Princeton University Press, 1983); Christine Leigh Heyrman, *Commerce and Culture: The Maritime Communities of Colonial Massachusetts, 1690–1750* (New York: Norton, 1984); and John Frederick Martin, *Profits in the Wilderness: Entrepreneurship and the Founding of New England Towns in the Seventeenth Century* (Chapel Hill: University of North Carolina Press, 1991). On the intersection of religion, gender, and politics in shaping communities, see Norton, *Founding Mothers and Fathers.*

45. Entry for April 2, 1677, in Thomas, ed., *Diary of Samuel Sewall*, vol. 1, p. 41.

46. Entries for January 2, 1701/02, and June 21, 1695, in ibid., pp. 459, 334–36; entry for July 17, 1726, in Walett, ed., *Diary of Ebenezer Parkman*, pp. 14–15.

47. Entry for July 17, 1726, in Walett, ed., *Diary of Ebenezer Parkman*, p. 15.

48. William Leete to John Winthrop Jr., June 22, 1658, in *Winthrop Papers*, pp. 540–41.

49. John Pynchon to John Winthrop Jr., June 24, 1667, in Carl Bridenbaugh, ed., *The Pynchon Papers*, vol. 1 (Boston: Colonial Society of Massachusetts, 1982), pp. 74–75.

50. Entry for January 12, 1746, in Wallet, ed., *Diary of Ebenezer Parkman*, p. 130.

51. Nathaniel Bouton, ed., *Documents and Records Relating to the Province of New Hampshire*, vol. 1 (Concord, N.H.: George E. Jenks, State Printer, 1867), pp 417–18.

52. 45-122 and 45-123, Essex County Court File Papers.

53. Ulrich, *A Midwife's Tale*, p. 149; for an example of this process in the seventeenth century, see the testimony of Elinor Baily, 15-128-1, Essex County Court File Papers.

54. 44-150-2, Essex County Court File Papers.

55. Natalie Zemon Davis, "Women on Top," in *Society and Culture in Early Modern France* (Stanford, Calif.: Stanford University Press, 1975), pp. 124–51; Cornelia Hughes Dayton, *Women before the Bar: Gender, Law, and Society in Connecticut, 1639–1789* (Chapel Hill: University of North Carolina Press, 1995), pp. 157–230.

56. 45-123-4, Essex County Court File Papers.

57. Testimony of Elizabeth Woostin, ibid.

58. Testimony of Goodwife Whicher, 45-122-1, Essex County Court File Papers.

59. Testimony of Dorothy Roberts, 45-122-3; and testimony of Marah Singletary, 45-123-3, Essex County Court File Papers.

60. Testimony of Michael Emmerson, 45-122-4; and confession of Robert Swan, 45-121-4, Essex County Court File Papers.

61. Testimony of Sara Davis, 45-124-3; and confession of Robert Swan, 45-121-4, Essex County Court File Papers.

62. Heyrman, *Commerce and Culture*, pp. 209–30.

63. Letter of John Bartoll, 8-66-1, Essex County Court File Papers.

64. Testimony of Mary Eburne, 8-70-1; and testimony of Mary Trevet, 8-69-1, Essex County Court File Papers.

65. Testimony of Elizabeth Legge, 8-70-2, Essex County Court File Papers.

66. Heyrman, *Commerce and Culture*, p. 227. On the leadership role of midwives and wealthy women, see Norton, *Founding Mothers and Fathers.*

67. 8-69-1, Essex County Court File Papers.

Chapter 4. A HIGHER CALLING

1. John Davenport to John Winthrop Jr., August 5, 1659, in Isabel Macbeath Calder, ed., *The Letters of John Davenport, Puritan Divine* (New Haven: Yale University Press, 1937), pp. 138–40.

2. Calder, "Introduction," in Calder, ed., *Letters of John Davenport*, pp. 1–12, quotation on p. 7.

3. A. Benedict Davenport, *A History and Genealogy of the Davenport Family in England and America, from A.D. 1086–1850* (New York: S. W. Benedict, 1851), p. 395.

4. Calder, "Introduction," p. 1; *Records of the Colony or Jurisdiction of New Haven from May 1653 to the Union* (Hartford, Conn.: Case, Lockwood, 1858), pp. 79, 306; *New Haven Town Records, 1649–1662*, vol.1 (New Haven: New Haven Colony Historical Society, 1917), pp. 272, 512, 100.

5. John Davenport to John Winthrop Jr., September 19, 1654, August 5, 1659, August 4, 1658, December 17, 1660, all in Calder, ed., *Letters of John Davenport*, pp. 97, 140, 127, 184.

6. See, for instance, the letter of August 5, 1659: "Many questions my wife hath. . . . Some she proposeth to send inclosed in this," in Calder, ed., *Letters of John Davenport*, p. 140.

7. Nicholas Culpeper, *Culpeper's Complete Herbal* (London: Milner, n.d.), p. 135; John Davenport to John Winthrop Jr., December 23, 1660, in Calder, ed., *Letters of John Davenport*, pp. 186–87. For a description of Elizabeth Davenport's skill at uroscopy, see chapter 1.

8. *Records of the Colony or Jurisdiction of New Haven*, p. 502.

9. Calder, ed., *Letters of John Davenport*, p. 137 n. 4, p. 189 n. 4; *New Haven Town Records, 1649–1662*, vol. 1, p. 510.

10. John Davenport to John Winthrop Jr., October 17, 1660, in Calder, ed., *Letters of John Daveport*, pp. 176–79.

11. John Davenport to John Winthrop Jr., August 6, 1659, ibid., p. 140.

12. John Davenport to John Winthrop Jr., August 4, 1658, and August 1, 1660, in ibid., pp. 127, 170.

13. Cotton Mather, *The Angel of Bethesda: An Essay upon the Common Maladies of Mankind*, ed. Gordon W. Jones (Barre, Mass.: American Antiquarian Society and Barre Publishers, 1972), p. 289.

14. Lucinda McCray Beier, *Sufferers and Healers: The Experience of Illness in Seventeenth-Century England* (London: Routledge and Kegan Paul, 1987), pp. 218–24; Linda Pollock, *With Faith and Physick: The Life of a Tudor Gentlewoman, Lady Grace Mildmay, 1552–1620* (London: Collins and Brown, 1993), pp. 110–42.

15. Pollock, *With Faith and Physick*, pp. 92–109, 102.

16. Patricia A. Watson, "The Hidden Ones: Women and Healing in Colonial New England," *Medicine and Healing: Annual Proceedings of the Dublin Seminar for New England Folklife* 15 (1990): 25–33.

17. S.[amuel?] Danforth to John Cotton Jr., March 3, 1687/88, Curwen Family Papers, Box One, Folder 4, American Antiquarian Society, Worcester, Mass.

18. Donald M. Scott, *From Office to Profession: The New England Ministry, 1750–1850* (Philadelphia: University of Pennsylvania Press, 1978), pp. 1–17.

19. John Willison, *The Afflicted Man's Companion: or, a directory for families afflicted with sickness, or any other distress* (Philadelphia: W. Young, Bookseller, 1788) (microfiche), p. 202; Benjamin Wadsworth, *Christian Advice to the sick and well* (Boston: J. Allen, Printer, 1714) (microfiche), p. 35. Both available at American Antiquarian Society, Worcester, Mass.

20. Micaiah Towgood, *Recovery from Sickness: a present to one lately raised from a dangerous disorder* (Boston: T. and J. Fleet, 1768) (microfiche), p. 24. Available at American Antiquarian Society, Worcester, Mass.

21. Pollock, *With Faith and Physick*, p. 108.

22. Robert C. Black, *The Younger John Winthrop* (New York: Columbia University Press, 1966), pp. 114–15. For more on Winthrop's education and status as an intellectual, see chapter 1.

23. Ibid., p. 156 (alchemical writings), p. 169 (Paracelsian influence).

24. Ibid., pp. 308–19.

25. Ibid., p. 170.

26. John Davenport to John Winthrop Jr., August 1, 1660, and August 4, 1658, in Calder, ed., *Letters of John Davenport*, pp. 170, 125.

27. John Davenport to John Winthrop Jr., August 4, 1658, and December 6, 1659, in ibid., pp. 126, 149.

28. Entry for February 1, 1663, in John Winthrop Jr., "Medical Records," Winthrop Papers, Massachusetts Historical Society, Boston (microfilm, Manuscripts and Archives, Yale University, New Haven, Conn.), vol. 2, p. 531; entry for April 21, 1666, in ibid., vol. 2, p. 647. Elizabeth Davenport also undertook nonmedical errands for Winthrop, such as hiring a servant for him and collecting his debts. See John Davenport's letters of November 22, 1655, and April 20, 1658, in Calder, ed., *Letters of John Davenport*, pp. 107–9, 120–21.

29. John Davenport to John Winthrop Jr., January 30, 1657/58, July 20, 1658, December 6, 1659, in ibid., pp. 113, 124, 150. This last quotation is a vivid example of Elizabeth's voice and presence in her husband's letters.

30. Culpeper, *Culpeper's Complete Herbal*, pp. 98–99; entry for January 5, 1660/61, in Winthrop, "Medical Records," vol. 1, p. 413.

31. Entries for December 29, and January 5, 1660/61, in ibid., vol. 1, p. 413.

32. Entry for February 18, 1661, in ibid., vol. 1, page number illegible. Like many of Winthrop's journal entries, this one is marred by blots and stains, and is made more difficult to read by Winthrop's idiosyncratic use of alchemical symbols. Given these limitations, I have done my best to transcribe Winthrop's words and decode his abbreviations and shorthand without misquoting or overinterpreting.

33. Gary Boyd Roberts, ed., *Genealogies of Connecticut Families*, vol. 2 (Baltimore: Genealogical Publishing, 1983), p. 513.

34. Entries for May 27 and June 4, 1658, in Winthrop, "Medical Records," vol. 1, p. 380.

35. Federal Writers' Project, *History of Milford Connecticut, 1639–1939* (Hartford, Conn.: Work Projects Administration for the State of Connecticut, 1939), pp. 8, 29.

36. Entry for January 10, 1667, in Winthrop, "Medical Records," vol. 2, p. 774.

37. John Davenport to John Winthrop Jr., December 23, 1660, and August 4, 1658, in Calder, ed., *Letters of John Davenport*, pp. 188, 27.

38. John Davenport to John Winthrop Jr., June 14, 1666, August, 1 1660, January 30, 1657/58, and December 10, 1659, in ibid., pp. 263, 170, 113, 148–49.

39. Gordon S. Wood, *The Radicalism of the American Revolution* (New York: Knopf, 1992), p. 38.

40. John Winthrop, *The History of New England* (Boston: Thomas V. Wait and Son, 1826), vol. 1, pp. 261–64.

41. David D. Hall, *Worlds of Wonder, Days of Judgment: Popular Religious Belief in Early New England* (Cambridge: Harvard University Press, 1989), pp. 71–116.

42. John Winthrop, *History of New England*, vol. 1, pp. 261–63, quotation on p. 261. Winthrop noted later in his journal that Jane Hawkins had long been suspected of witchcraft, both in Massachusetts and in England.

43. John Cotton, "The Way of the Congregational Churches Cleared," in David D. Hall, ed., *The Antinomian Controversy, 1636–1638: A Documentary History* (Middletown, Conn.: Wesleyan University Press, 1968), pp. 397–437, quotation on 411–12.

44. John Winthrop, "A Short Story of the Rise, reign, and ruine of the Antinomians, Familists, & Libertines," in Hall, ed., *Antinomian Controversy*, pp. 201–310, quotation on p. 263.

45. Ibid., p. 264.

46. "Examination of Mrs. Anne Hutchinson at the Court at Newtown," in Hall, ed., *Antinomian Controversy*, pp. 312–48.

47. Philip F. Gura, *A Glimpse of Sion's Glory: Puritan Radicalism in New England, 1620–1660* (Middletown, Conn.: Wesleyan University Press, 1984), pp. 237–75; Edmund S. Morgan, "The Case against Anne Hutchinson," in Francis J. Bremer, ed., *Anne Hutchinson: Troubler of the Puritan Zion* (Huntington, N.Y.: Krieger Publishing, 1981), pp. 51–58; Mary Beth Norton, *Founding Mothers and Fathers: Gendered Power and the Forming of American Society* (New York: Knopf, 1996), pp. 359–400.

48. Norton, *Founding Mothers and Fathers*, pp. 360–69.

49. "A Report of the Trial of Mrs. Anne Hutchinson before the Church in Boston," in Hall, ed., *Antinomian Controversy*, pp. 350–88, quotation on 370.

Chapter 5. CALLED TO COURT

1. 15-128-1, Essex County Court File Papers, Essex Institute, Salem, Mass. (microfilm, Yale University, New Haven, Conn.).

2. A. G. Roeber, "Authority, Law and Custom: The Rituals of Court Day in Tidewater Virginia, 1720–1750," *William and Mary Quarterly,* 3rd series, 37 (1980): 29–52; Rhys Isaac, *The Transformation of Virginia, 1740–1790* (New York: Norton, 1982), pp. 88–94; David Thomas Konig, *Law and Society in Puritan Massachusetts: Essex County, 1629–1692* (Chapel Hill: University of North Carolina Press, 1979).

3. Roeber, "Authority, Law and Custom," pp. 37–38, 51.

4. Ibid.; Konig, *Law and Society*.

5. Cornelia Hughes Dayton, *Women before the Bar: Law, Gender, and Society in Connecticut, 1639–1789* (Chapel Hill: University of North Carolina Press, 1995), pp. 30–33.

6. This description of court day in York, Maine, comes from the detailed description in Neil Allen Jr., "Law and Authority to the Eastward: Maine Courts, Magistrates, and Lawyers, 1690–1730," in Daniel R. Coquillette, ed., *Law in Colonial Massachusetts, 1630–1800* (Boston: Colonial Society of Massachusetts, 1984), pp. 290–311. On the gendered nature of legal proceedings, see Mary Beth Norton, *Founding Mothers and Fathers: Gendered Power and the Forming of American Society* (New York: Knopf, 1996).

7. Dayton, *Women before the Bar*, pp. 15–17.

8. Testimony of John Dole, 22-84-1, Essex County Court File Papers.

9. Testimony of Philip Reade, 1671/2-60-4, Middlesex County Court Files (microfilm), Massachusetts State Archives, Columbia Point, Boston.

10. *New Haven Town Records, 1649–1662*, vol. 1 (New Haven: New Haven Colony Historical Society, 1917), pp. 97–98, 265, 67, 80.

11. Ibid., vol. 2, pp. 184–85.

12. *Records and Files of the Quarterly Courts of Essex County*, vol. 2 (Salem, Mass.: Essex Institute, 1911), p. 119.

13. C. L'Estrange Ewen, *Witchcraft and Demonianism* (London: Heath Cranton, 1933), p. 75.

14. Ibid., p. 250.

15. David D. Hall, ed. *Witch-Hunting in Seventeenth-Century New England: A Documentary History, 1638–1692* (Boston: Northeastern University Press, 1991), p. 216.

16. Testimony of Elizabeth Rinke, Docket #257, Suffolk County Court Files (microfilm), Massachusetts Archives, Columbia Point, Boston.

17. *The First Laws of the Commonwealth of Massachusetts* (Wilmington, Del.: Michael Glazier, 1981), p. 246.

18. On the special trust in women's word, see Dayton, *Women before the Bar*, pp. 31–32; on the persistence of the childbirth "examination," see Laurel Thatcher Ulrich, *A Midwife's Tale: The Life of Martha Ballard Based on Her Diary, 1785–1812* (New York: Knopf, 1990), pp. 147–60. This practice may soon be revived. In a recent National Public Radio piece on new programs to collect child support from unwed fathers, a delivery-room nurse stated that the easiest way to coax a woman to name the father of her child was to ask during labor.

19. 38-4-1, Essex County Court File Papers.

20. Testimony of Grace Duch, 6-16-3, Essex County Court File Papers.

21. See, for example, Paul Boyer and Stephen Nissenbaum, *Salem Possessed: The Social Origins of Witchcraft* (Cambridge: Harvard University Press, 1974); and John Putnam Demos, *Entertaining Satan: Witchcraft and the Culture of Early New England* (New York: Oxford University Press, 1982), pp. 213–314.

22. Christine Leigh Heyrman, *Commerce and Culture: The Maritime Communities of Colonial Massachusetts, 1690–1750* (New York: Norton, 1984), pp. 34–41.

23. Testimony of William Vincent, 3-108-1, Essex County Court File Papers.

24. Feeling the belly, removing name from "paper," Browne's curses, testimony of Margaret Prince, 3-110-8, Essex County Court File Papers; Mrs. Millet, testimony of Goodwife Parkman, 3-111-1, Essex County Court File Papers.

25. Testimony of "the wife of John Mattell," 3-111-2, Essex County Court File Papers; testimony of Isabel Babson, 3-113-1, Essex County Court File Papers.

26. Testimony of Grace Duch, Elinor Baily, Joane Collens, and Sarra Vinson, 3-109-1, Essex County Court File Papers.

27. Testimony of Isabel Babson, 3-113-1, Essex County Court File Papers.

28. Ibid.

29. Testimony of Mary Millet, 3-108-3, Essex County Court File Papers.

30. Testimony of Isabel Babson, 3-113-1, Essex County Court File Papers.

31. Heyrman, *Commerce and Culture*, p. 41.

32. Testimony of Elinor Baily, 38-18-2, Essex County Court File Papers.

33. *New Haven Town Records*, vol. 1, p. 96.

34. Docket #1254, Suffolk County Court Files. During the early colonial period, a woman's word was given more weight than her alleged attacker's; in the early eighteenth century, there was a much more skeptical attitude on the part of magistrates and juries, and a reluctance to convict. This case appears to be transitional: the jury finds Peter Croy guilty, but only after they are convinced that the two-

witness rule has been technically satisfied. For a detailed discussion of New England rape prosecutions, see Dayton, *Women before the Bar*, pp. 231–84.

35. Case of Thomas Keeney and Ciceley Indian, 1678-80-2, Middlesex County Court Files.

36. Case of Elizabeth Pierce and Benjamin Simons, 1677-71-3, Middlesex County Court Files.

37. 1-106-1, Essex County Court File Papers.

38. 38-4-1, Essex County Court File Papers.

39. Testimony of Elizabeth Brewster, in *Records of the Colony or Jurisdiction of New Haven from May 1653 to the Union* (Hartford, Conn.: Case Lockwood, 1858), pp. 81–82.

40. Ibid.

41. Testimony of Goodwife Thompson, *Records of the Colony or Jurisdiction of New Haven*, p. 84.

42. Konig, *Law and Society*, pp. 150–57.

43. Testimony of John Dole, 34-95-2, Essex County Court File Papers.

44. Testimony of John Paul, 11-49-2, Essex County Court File Papers. Chapter 5 examines Ann Edmonds's career at length.

45. Testimony of Sarah Hill, 11-60-2, Essex County Court File Papers.

46. Testimony of Thomas Browne, 11-60-4, Essex County Court File Papers.

47. Ibid.

48. See Konig, *Law and Society*, for other ways courts regulated who could and could not become part of a community.

49. 37-73-4, Essex County Court File Papers.

50. Testimony of Elinor Baily, 15-128-1, Essex County Court File Papers.

51. Ibid.

52. Lucinda McCray Beier, *Sufferers and Healers: The Experience of Illness in Seventeenth-Century England* (London: Routledge and Kegan Paul, 1987), p. 15.

53. Quoted in ibid., p. 18.

54. Carol Karlsen, *The Devil in the Shape of a Woman: Witchcraft in Colonial New England* (New York: Norton, 1987).

55. *Aristotle's Compleat Masterpiece: In Three Parts: Displaying the secrets of nature in the generation of man. Regularly digested in chapters and sections, rendering it far more useful and easy than any yet extant*, 26th ed. ([London?]: Printed and Sold by the Booksellers, 1755), p. 62.

56. 38-18-2, Essex County Court File Papers.

57. Case of John Garland and Dow, Docket #1412, Suffolk County Court Files.

58. Londa Schiebinger, *The Mind Has No Sex? Women in the Origins of Modern Science* (Cambridge: Harvard University Press, 1989); and "Skeletons in the Closet: The First Illustrations of the Female Skeleton in Eighteenth-Century Anatomy," in Thomas Laqueur and Catherine Gallagher, eds., *The Making of the Modern Body: Sexuality and Society in the Nineteenth Century* (Berkeley: University of California Press, 1987), pp. 42–82. Ian Maclean discusses the relationship between scholarly ideas about women's bodies and social ideas about women's place at length in *The Renaissance Notion of Woman: A Study in the Fortunes of Scholasticism and Medical Science in European Intellectual Life* (New York: Cambridge University Press, 1980). Maclean writes that the ancient concept of women's bodies as imperfect men's bodies was fading in the seventeenth century, but the idea that women were less worthy of study was not. Maclean notes that while anatomists such as William Harvey made studies of women and female reproductive anatomy, their

work was "indeed important, but more to posterity than to contemporaries" (p. 37).

Chapter 6. CALLING THE DOCTORESS

1. Entries for March 22 and March 31, 1760, in Diary of Ebenezer Parkman, 1756–1761, Parkman Family Papers, American Antiquarian Society, Worcester, Mass.

2. Entry for January 23, 1774, in "Diary of Mary Viall Holyoke," in George Francis Dow, ed., *The Holyoke Diaries* (Salem: Essex Institute, 1911) (microfilm), p. 82; entry for April 3, 1677, in M. Halsey Thomas, ed., *The Diary of Samuel Sewall*, vol. 1 (New York: Farrar, Straus and Giroux, 1973), p. 41.

3. Entry for July 25, 1758, in Diary of Ebenezer Parkman, Parkman Family Papers.

4. Entry for April 2, 1677, in Thomas, ed., *Diary of Samuel Sewall*, vol. 1, p. 41; 1678-82-3, Middlesex County Court Files (microfilm), Massachusetts Archives, Columbia Point, Boston.

5. 38-5-2, 38-3-3, and 38-4-2, Essex County Court File Papers, Essex Institute, Salem, Mass. (microfilm, Yale University, New Haven, Conn.).

6. 36-78-2, Essex County Court File Papers.

7. Entries for April 2–15, 1759, in Diary of Ebenezer Parkman, Parkman Family Papers.

8. 11-59-2, Essex County Court File Papers.

9. Entry for March 25, 1760, in Diary of Ebenezer Parkman, Parkman Family Papers.

10. *Records and Files of the Quarterly Courts of Essex County*, vol. 6 (Salem: Essex Institute, 1911), p. 38.

11. Will of Frances Hawes, in ibid., vol. 1, p. 86; inventory of John Bread, in ibid., vol. 6, p. 134.

12. Entries for April 1–3, 1677, in Thomas, ed., *Diary of Samuel Sewall*, vol. 1, pp. 41–42.

13. Entries for December 21–24, 1685, in ibid., pp. 89–90.

14. 2-106-1 and 2-130-1, Essex County Court File Papers.

15. Entry for October 14, 1758, in Diary of Ebenezer Parkman, Parkman Family Papers.

16. Inventory of Henry Sewall, in *Records and Files of the Quarterly Courts of Essex County*, vol. 1, p. 419.

17. Ibid., vol. 5, pp. 402–3. Hoyt may have come to regret her practice, however—Tewksbury was soon charged with "unseemly carriages" with Hoyt's married daughter, Mary Marten.

18. 12-136-1 and 20-41-3, Essex County Court File Papers.

19. Nancy Siraisi, *Medieval and Early Renaissance Medicine: An Introduction to Knowledge and Practice* (Chicago: University of Chicago Press, 1990), pp. 13, 27. On Trotula, Siraisi notes that while her existence has been questioned, the evidence indicates that she probably was a real woman who wrote a general medical treatise, although the midwifery text attributed to her is probably spurious.

20. Alice Clark, *Working Life of Women in the Seventeenth Century*, new ed. (London: Routledge and Kegan Paul, 1982), p. 265.

21. Lucinda McCray Beier, *Sufferers and Healers: The Experience of Illness in Seventeenth-Century England* (London: Routledge and Kegan Paul, 1987), pp. 8–50.

22. Entry for May 7, 1666, in Increase Mather Diary Typescript, Folder 1, Mather Family Papers, American Antiquarian Society, Worcester, Mass., transcription by Michael Hall, p. 110; 33-67-2, Essex County Court File Papers.

23. Testimony of Mary Hale, 33-67-2, Essex County Court File Papers.

24. Ibid.

25. Ibid.

26. Testimony of Hannah Mann, 33-68-1, Essex County Court File Papers.

27. Testimony of Mary Hale, 33-67-2, Essex County Court File Papers.

28. Ibid.

29. *Records and Files of the Quarterly Courts of Essex County*, vol. 5, p. 405.

30. See, for example, the case of the stranger with the plague, discussed in chapter 5.

31. Testimony of Brigid Huggins, 5-141-3, Essex County Court File Papers.

32. Testimony of Joseph Edmonds, 5-139-4, Essex County Court File Papers.

33. 5-141-1, Essex County Court File Papers.

34. 5-134-1, Essex County Court File Papers.

35. Testimony of Joseph Edmonds, 5-139-4, Essex County Court File Papers.

36. Testimony of Sarah Jenkens, 5-143-3, Essex County Court File Papers.

37. Testimony of Giles Fifield, 5-142-3, Essex County Court File Papers.

38. Testimony of Matthew Price, 5-137-3, Essex County Court File Papers.

39. Testimony of Anthony Crosbee, 5-141-1, Essex County Court File Papers.

40. Testimony of Robert Tuck, 5-146-4, Essex County Court File Papers.

41. Testimony of Sarah Jenkens, 5-143-3, Essex County Court File Papers.

42. Testimony of Thomas Marshall, 5-143-3, Essex County Court File Papers.

43. Testimony of Giles Fifield, 5-142-3, Essex County Court File Papers.

44. Entry for July 9, 1756, in Diary of Ebenezer Parkman, Parkman Family Papers. Mrs. Kimball's medicine was apparently effective—Parkman recorded that it allowed him to eat "with relish" for the first time in days.

45. Sore breast, in 27-43-1, Essex County Court File Papers; Banfield, in *Records and Files of the Quarterly Courts of Essex County*, vol. 6, p. 301.

46. Andrew V. Rapoza, "The Trials of Phillip Reade, Seventeenth-Century Itinerant Physician," *Annual Proceedings of the Dublin Seminar for New England Folklife* 15 (1990): 82–94.

47. Reade vs. Parker, 1673-62-5, Middlesex County Court Files. Reade was not always so successful—he lost another debt case when the defendants successfully claimed that "he never gave but tow porshions of Phisick." See Reade vs. Langdon, 1695-197-3, Middlesex County Court Files.

48. John Putnam Demos, *Entertaining Satan: Witchcraft and the Culture of Early New England* (New York: Oxford University Press, 1982), p. 84.

49. Docket #1972, Suffolk County Court Files (microfilm), Massachusetts Archives, Columbia Point, Boston.

50. Testimony of Hannah Weacome, Docket #1972, Suffolk County Court Files. Richard Godbeer includes a discussion of this case in *The Devil's Dominion: Magic and Religion in Early New England* (New York: Cambridge University Press, 1992), pp. 45–46.

51. Testimony of Margaret Ellis, Docket #1972, Suffolk County Court Files.

52. *Records of the Court of Assistants of the Colony of the Massachusetts Bay 1630–1692*, vol. 1 (Boston: County of Suffolk, 1901), p. 11.

53. David D. Hall, *Witch-Hunting in Seventeenth-Century New England: A Documentary History, 1638–1692* (Boston: Northeastern University Press, 1991), p. 249.

54. Testimony of Esther Wilson, in ibid., pp. 246–47; testimony of Jane Sewall, in ibid., pp. 249–50.

55. "the divill take you . . . ," in Rapoza, "The Trials of Phillip Reade," p. 89; also quoted in David D. Hall, *Worlds of Wonder, Days of Judgment: Popular Religious Belief in Colonial New England* (Cambridge: Harvard University Press, 1989), p. 294; "knok out the Doktor's brains," in 1668-48-2, Middlesex County Court Files.

56. Reade vs. Hill, 1669-49-2, Middlesex County Court Files.

57. The documents in this case are reprinted in Hall, ed., *Witch-Hunting*, pp. 185–88; Reade's testimony is on p. 186.

58. Ibid., p. 185.

59. Jane Kamensky, "Female Speech and Other Demons: Witchcraft and Word-craft in Early New England," in Elizabeth Reis, ed., *Spellbound: Women and Witch-craft in America* (Wilmington, Del.: Scholarly Resources, 1998), pp. 53–74.

60. Demos, *Entertaining Satan*, appendix, pp. 401–9. The healers on Demos's list are Jane Hawkins, Anne Hutchinson, Margaret Jones, Grace Duch, Elizabeth Garlick, Winifred Holman, Katherine Harrison, Ann Burt, Ann Edmonds, Elizabeth Morse, Mary Hale, Rachel Fuller, and Hannah Jones.

61. Such anomalous positions, such as owning large tracts of land, often made women vulnerable to witchcraft accusations. See Carol Karlsen, *The Devil in the Shape of a Woman: Witchcraft in Colonial New England* (New York: Norton, 1987).

62. Testimony of John Gibson, in Hall, ed., *Witch-Hunting*, pp. 135–43, quotations on p. 135.

63. 1663-34-2, Middlesex County Court Files.

64. Hall, *Witch-Hunting*, pp. 144–45, quotation on p. 145.

Epilogue

1. Entries for August 17–25, 1752, in Francis G. Walett, ed., *The Diary of Ebenezer Parkman, 1703–1782* (Worcester, Mass.: American Antiquarian Society, 1974), pp. 259–60.

2. For a discussion of the changes in law and commerce, see Cornelia Hughes Dayton, *Women before the Bar: Gender, Law, and Society in Connecticut, 1639–1789* (Chapel Hill: University of North Carolina Press, 1995).

3. Entry for December 7, 1758, in Diary of Ebenezer Parkman, 1756–1761, Parkman Family Papers, American Antiquarian Society, Worcester, Mass.

4. Eric Christianson, "The Medical Practitioners of Massachusetts, 1630–1800: Patterns of Change and Continuity," in J. Worth Estes, ed., *Medicine in Colonial Massachusetts, 1620–1820* (Boston: Colonial Society of Massachusetts, 1980), pp. 49–68.

5. Entries for April 2–29, 1759, in Diary of Ebenezer Parkman, Parkman Family Papers; quotations from entry for April 15.

6. John C. Greene, "The Boston Medical Community and Emerging Science, 1780–1820," in Estes, ed., *Medicine in Colonial Massachusetts*, pp. 187–97.

7. Richard D. Brown, "The Healing Arts in Colonial and Revolutionary Massachusetts: The Context for Scientific Medicine," in Estes, ed., *Medicine in Colonial Massachusetts*, pp. 35–47.

8. Obituary of Benjamin Gott, *Boston Gazette or Weekly Journal*, July 30, 1751. A similar item ran in *Boston Weekly Newsletter*, August 1, 1751.

9. Entry for March 19, 1737, in Walett, ed., *Diary of Ebenezer Parkman*, pp. 40, 41 n. 6.

10. Entries for February 20–28, 1738, and July 24, 1738, in ibid., pp. 45, 49.

11. Entry for August 10, 1738, in ibid., p. 50.

12. Entries for December 16–28, 1738, in ibid., pp. 55–56.

13. Ibid.

14. Dayton, *Women before the Bar*, pp. 69–79. Dayton notes, however, that commercial relationships grew more impersonal as the eighteenth century went on.

15. My thanks to Professor Ross Beales of the College of the Holy Cross, who performed the computer searches that provided this information.

16. Entry for March 22, 1760, in Diary of Ebenezer Parkman, Parkman Family Papers.

17. Entries for April 2–29, 1759, in ibid.

18. Entry for October 4, 1725, in Wallet, ed., *Diary of Ebenezer Parkman*, p. 7; entries for February 1–9, 1758, and July 30–August 2, 1758, in Diary of Ebenezer Parkman, Parkman Family Papers.

19. Jane B. Donegan, "'Safe Delivered,' but by Whom? Midwives and Men-Midwives in Early America," and Catherine M. Scholten, "On the Importance of the Obstetrick Art: Changing Customs of Childbirth in America, 1760–1825," in Judith Walzer Leavitt, ed., *Women and Health in America* (Madison: University of Wisconsin Press, 1984), pp. 302–17, 142–54; Judith Walzer Leavitt, *Brought to Bed: Childbearing in America, 1750–1950* (New York: Oxford University Press, 1986).

20. Brown, "The Healing Arts," p. 41; *The Husbandman's Guide, in Four Parts* (New York: William and Andrew Bradford, Printers, 1712), copy at American Antiquarian Society (AAS), Worcester, Mass.

21. See, for example, the following book catalogues from the AAS: *The Library of the late Reverend and Learned Mr. Samuel Lee . . .* (Boston: Printed by Benjamin Harris for Duncan Campbell, bookseller, 1693); *A Catalogue of curious and valuable books, belonging to the late reverend and learned Mr. Ebenezer Pemberton . . .* (Boston: Printed by B. Green and may be had gratis at the shop of Samuel Gerrish, bookseller, 1717); *A Catalogue of Books, in all Arts and Sciences to be sold at the shop of T. Cox, bookseller . . .* (Boston: T. Cox, 1734); *A Catalogue of Books, imported and to be sold by Henry Knox . . .* (Boston: Henry Knox, 1772).

22. Entry for December 13, 1760, in Diary of Ebenezer Parkman, Parkman Family Papers.

23. Nathaniel Williams, *The Method of Practice in the Small-Pox, with Observations on the Way of Inoculation* (Boston: Printed and Sold by S. Kneeland, 1752), first page of preface (unnumbered).

24. Ibid., title page.

25. Entries for May 14, 1770, November 22, 1771, November 21, 1770, and March 25–April 5, 1777, in "Diary of Mary Viall Holyoke," in George Francis Dow, ed., *The Holyoke Diaries* (Salem: Essex Institute, 1911), pp. 73, 77, 95.

26. Entries for January 8–14, 1764, and January 20–23, 1774, in "Diary of Mary Viall Holyoke," pp. 60, 81–82.

27. Richard Hall Wiswell, "Doctor Edward Augustus Holyoke," in *Sketches about Salem People* (Salem: The Club, 1930), pp. 6–21.

28. Entries for October 11–31, 1768 (Mrs. Oliver and Mrs. Lynde); February 9, 1765, and July 5, 1769 (Mrs. Browne); April 6, 1763, and October 31, 1768 (Molly and Nathaniel Appleton), in "Diary of Mary Viall Holyoke," pp. 58, 70.

29. Laurel Thatcher Ulrich, *Good Wives: Image and Reality in the Lives of Women in Northern New England, 1650–1750* (New York: Oxford University Press, 1990), pp. 68–86; Carol Berkin, *First Generations: Women in Colonial America* (New York:

Hill and Wang, 1996); entry for April 28, 1784, in "Diary of Mary Viall Holyoke," p. 111.

30. Entries for March 10, 1758, and March 22, 1760, in Diary of Ebenezer Parkman, Parkman Family Papers; Laurel Thatcher Ulrich, *A Midwife's Tale: The Life of Martha Ballard Based on Her Diary, 1785–1812* (New York: Knopf, 1990).

31. Ulrich, *Midwife's Tale*, pp. 235–61.

32. Ibid., pp. 178–79, 254–55, 251.

33. Ibid., pp. 147–61.

34. For a more general discussion of changes in fornication and paternity cases, see Dayton, *Women before the Bar*, pp. 157–230.

35. Harriot K. Hunt, *Glances and Glimpses; or Fifty Years Social, Including Twenty Years Professional Life* (Boston: John P. Jewett, 1856).

36. Ibid., p. 122.

37. Ibid., p. 108.

38. Ibid., pp. 108–9.

39. Ibid., p. 119.

40. Ibid., p. 250.

41. Ibid.

42. Ibid., p. 252.

43. Regina Markell Morantz-Sanchez, *Sympathy and Science: Women Physicians in American Medicine* (New York: Oxford University Press, 1985), p. 188.

44. Elizabeth Blackwell, *Pioneer Work in Opening the Medical Profession to Women* (London: Longmans, Green, 1895), p. 30.

45. Ibid., pp. 254, 27.

46. For a thorough discussion of Blackwell's career and her views of womanhood and politics, see Morantz-Sanchez, *Sympathy and Science.*

Index

Numbers in italics refer to illustrations

Brigham, Samuel, 13
Brigham women's medical notebook, 8,
	17–19, *18*, 23–24, 41
	abortion, 36–37, *38*
	hemorrhoids cure, 7–8
	remedy for threatened miscarriage, 32
Brown, Antoinette, 151
Brown, Richard, 143
Browne, Ebenezer, 28, 109–10
Browne, Thomas, 108–9
Browne, William, 100–103
Burt, Ann, 130

Calder, Isabel, 72
Calling the women together, 45, 60–61
Callings, xv–xvi
Carr, George, 103, 112
Chaise, Dr., 97
Chase, Ann, 93, 110
Chase, Dr., 9, 138
Chater, Alice, 117
Chater, John, 117
Cheaver, Esther, 104
Childbirth
	ceremonies following, xi, 48, 115, 146
	exclusion of men from, 8, 47, 48
	gathering of women for, 45–50
	and physicians, 141, 143
	scenarios, xi, xii, 34–36, 45, 93
	and sex role reversal, 63–64
	test for determining paternity, xii–xiii,
		63, 93, 98–100, 105, 110, 147–48,
		166 n. 18
Children, abandoned, 115
Cole, Ann, 57, 59
Cole, Eunice, 98
Coleman, Dr., 147
Colostrum, 36
Comfrey, 80
Competition among healers, 123–24,
	130–31
Cooper, Goodwife, 32
Cotton, Dorothy, 76, 154 n. 21
Cotton, John, 84, 86, 87–88
Court hand (handwriting style), 20
Courts of law
	debt cases, 121–24, 125
	masculinity of, 93–94, 95–96
	men's versus women's roles, 97–98
	paternity suits, xii–xiii, 63–67, 93,
		98–100, 105, 110, 147–48, 166 n. 18
	rape trials, 103–4, 167 n. 34
	respect for healers, 96–97

slander suits, 130, 132–33
social rituals of, 95–98
See also Witchcraft trials
Cromwell, Anna, 22
Crosbee, Anthony, 123
Crosby, Dr., 138, 141
Croy, Peter, 104, 166–67 n. 34
Culpeper, Nicholas, 5

Davenport, Benedict, 72
Davenport, Bridget, 115
Davenport, Elizabeth
	cooperation with John Winthrop Jr.,
		xiv, 71, 72–75, 78–81, 83, 88,
		164 n. 28
	diagnostic skills, 28, 29, 73–74, 80
	knowledge of household medicine,
		26, 73
	medical network of, 74, 77, 78
	and uroscopy, 29, 73–74, 80
	See also Gentlewomen healers;
		Women healers
Davenport, John, 71, 72–73, 79–80, 82–83
Davenport, John, Jr., 49
Davis, Goodwife, 65
Davis, Sara, 63–64, 65–67
Deafness, cure for, 40
Debt cases, 121–24, 125
Demos, John, 126, 132
Digby, Sir Kenelm, 41
Digby's Closet, 19, 143
Disease
	classification of, 5
	theories of, 15–16
Distillings, herbal, 27, 156 n. 14
Doctoresses, 118–33
	authority of, 119, 124
	compared with other healers, 114–15,
		118, 124–25, 131
	cooperation with physicians,
		121–22, 123
	fees of, 118, 120, 122, 125
	history of, 119
	witchcraft accusations against,
		125–29, 130–33
	See also Edmonds, Ann; Hale, Mary;
		Women healers
Doctors. *See* Physicians
Doctrine of similars, 6
Dole, Goodwife, xii, xiii
Dole, John, 12, 96, 112, 113
Dounton, Rebeckah, 116–17
Drury, Mary, 48–49

Duch, Grace, 99–100, 102, 105
Dunlop, Patty, 115, 116

Eaton, Theophilus, 72
Eburne, Mary, 68
Edmonds, Ann, 107–9, 111–12, 119,
    121–24, 125
  witchcraft accusations against,
    127–28, 132
  See also Doctoresses
Edmonds, William, 108, 121–22
Ela, Daniel, 12
Elderflowers, 26–27
Ellis, Margaret, 126, 127
Emetics, 6, 33
Enemas, 6
England, ties with New England, 135–36
English Housewife, The (Markham), 26

Fairechild, Mrs., 49, 77
Fees
  doctoresses', 118, 120, 122, 125
  midwives', 125
  nurses', 116–17
Fifield, Giles, 124
Folklore
  bleeding of body in presence of mur-
    derer, 57, 102
  deformed children, 85
  laying of scarlet cloth, 115
  swallows, 41–42
  truth-telling during childbirth,
    xii–xiii, 63, 93, 98–100, 105, 110,
    147–48
Folsham, Mary, 121
Forbes, Thomas Rogers, 15
Forbush, Dorcas ("Granny"), 45, 53, 54,
    61, 139
Forceps, 141
Fornication, 39, 64, 66, 97, 112, 147–48
Fox, Ann, 116
Fuller, Rachel, 42–43, 44, 62

Galenic humoral medicine, 4–6, 33
Garland, John, 112–13
Gatchell, John, 69
Gatchell, Wiboro, 68–69, 105
Gender
  and authority of science, 112–13
  and literacy, 19–21
  in medical practice, xiv, 12, 14–15,
    81–82
  and witchcraft accusations, 131

Gender ambiguity, 110–11
Gender hierarchy, 12, 110–11
Geneva Medical College, 151
Gentlewomen healers, 75–76, 118. *See
    also* Davenport, Elizabeth; Hutchin-
    son, Ann
Gibbs, Mistress, 120
Gibson, John, 132
Glances and Glimpses (Hunt), 149
Gloucester, Mass., 100–103
Glover, Goodwife, 105
Godfrey, Goodwife, 42–43
Goite, Peter, 105
Goodyear, Mrs., 74
Gossip. *See* Medical gatherings,
    women's
Gott, Benjamin, 139–40
Green, Henry, 122, 123
Green, Mary, 122–23
Greenslet, Widow, 107
Greensmith, Nathaniel, 59
Greensmith, Rebecca, 56, 59

Hale, Mary, 119–21, 124, 125
  witchcraft accusations against,
    126–27, 132
  See also Doctoresses
Halfway covenant, 55
Handwriting as marker of social status,
    20–21
Harrison, Katherine, 57–58, 161 n. 39
Hartford Controversy, 55
Hartford witch-hunt, 55–60, 161 n. 39
Harvard Medical College, 149
Harvesting of medicinal herbs, 26
Harvey, William, 4, 167–68 n. 58
Harwood, Rachel, 48–49
Hawkins, Dr., 121
Hawkins, Jane, 85
Hazen, Hannah, 110
Healers, 12–14, 96–97
  authority of, 97–98, 103
  categories of, 6–7, 8, 9–14
  cooperation among, 12, 14, 61, 136,
    147
  medical records compared, 15–20
  relationship with patients, 6
  role of gender, xiv, 12, 14–15, 81–82
  See also Doctoresses; Housewives;
    Midwives; Physicians; Women
    healers
Healy, Grace, 104
Hemingway, Dr., 141

and women's social networks, xi,
50–51
See also Women's communities
Medical hierarchy, xiv, 9–14, 110–11
Medical practitioners. *See* Healers
Medical schools, xv, 149, 151–52
Medical societies, 16–17, 138
Medicine, x, 3–8
    academic, 138, 143
    Galenic paradigm, 4–6, 33
    lay versus learned, 3, 7–8
    Paracelsian paradigm, 5–6
Medicines
    preparation of, 24, 26–28
    as preventive measures, 33
Menstruation, obstructed, 37–38, 80–81.
    See also Abortion; Miscarriages
*Method and Practice in the Small-Pox with
    Observations on the way of Inocula-
    tion, The* (Williams), 143–44
Midwives, xv, 8, 32, 96–97
    advocacy by, 93–94, 100
    authority of, xii–xiii, 97–98, 103–7,
        111–13, 148
    compared with doctoresses, 124–25
    double role of, 109–10, 112
    enforcement of social norms, xii–xiii,
        107–9
    gender ambiguity of, 110–11
    role in paternity suits, xii–xiii, 63, 93,
        98–100, 105, 110, 147–48
    See also Childbirth; Witchcraft trials;
        Women healers
Miggat, Goodwife, 58
Mildmay, Lady Grace, 75–76
Millet, Mrs., 101
Millet, Thomas, 101, 102
Miscarriages, 32, 37–38. *See also* Abor-
    tion; Menstruation, obstructed
Moores, Constance, xii
Morse, Elizabeth, 128–29, 132
Mothers, questioning of unwed, xii–xiii,
    63, 93, 98–100, 105, 110, 147–48,
    166 n. 18
Mott, Mrs., 149
*Mr. Watson's Essay on Fevers, the Rattles
    and Canker*, 143

Native Americans, 19
New England, ties with England, 135–36
New Haven Colony, 71, 72, 74–75, 83
    witchcraft trials, 105–6
Newman, Francis, 74

Newton, Mrs. Roger, 81, 82, 88
Newton, Roger, 82
Nurses, 114–18

Oakes, Dr., xi
Opium, 141
Ormsby, Richard, 98
Orphans, 115

Palmer, Thomas, 7–8, 15, 16, 17
Paracelsian medicine, 5–6
Paracelsus, 4
Parker, Mrs., 114, 140, 146
Parkman, Ebenezer, 13, 14, 62, 114, 116
    and barter economy, 54–55
    on bloodletting, 8–9
    shift in preference toward physicians,
        137–38, 139–41
    and women's medical gatherings, 45,
        48, 49, 60, 61
Parkman, Hannah Breck, 31, 45, 135
    use of nurses, 115, 116
    use of physicians, 139, 140, 141, 143
    and women's community, 52–55
Parkman, Molly Champney, 32, 52–53,
    61
Parks, Mary Brigham, 23
Parling, Goodwife, 115
Paternity suits, xii–xiii, 63–67, 93,
    98–100, 105, 110, 147–48, 166 n. 18
Patients, relationship with healers, 6
Perkins, William, 101, 102, 107
Physicians
    authority of, 96, 112
    and childbirth, 141, 143
    and doctoresses, 121–22, 123, 131
    dominance in eighteenth century, xv,
        136–41
    education of, 136, 138
    empiric, 7, 11–12
    learned, ix–x, 7, 10–11
    redefinition in eighteenth century,
        135–37
    women, xv, 148, 151–52
    See also Healers
Pickling, 26–27
Pierce, Elizabeth, 104
*Pioneer Work in Opening the Medical
    Profession to Women* (Blackwell), 152
Plague, 108
Plants, medicinal, 26–28
Potter, Hannah, 97
Potter, Rebeckah, 97

Williams, Nathaniel, 143–44
Williams, Ruth, 105, 115–16
Williams, Thomas, 62
Willis, Dr., 138, 141
Wills, 103
Wilmott, Sarah, 81
Wilson, Alice, 128
Winchester, Elizabeth Champney, 52
Winthrop, John, Jr., 15, 49, 62
    claims to gentility, 10–11, 20, 83–84
    cooperation with Elizabeth Daven-
        port, xiv, 71, 72–75, 78–81, 83, 88,
        164 n. 28
    education of, 10–11, 77–78
    medical network of, 81–82
    medical theories of, 5, 16, 78
    member of Royal Society, 17, 78
Winthrop, John, Sr., 10, 84, 85, 86
Witchcraft trials, xiii–xiv
    of doctoresses, 125–29, 130–33
    in Gloucester, Mass., 100–103
    in Hartford, Conn., 55–60, 161 n. 39
    interest of men in, 58–59
    in New Haven Colony, 105–6
    of Rachel Fuller, 42–43, 44, 62
    and swimming test, 59
    use of searchers, 97–98
    See also Courts of law
Witches, image of, xiii
Women
    anatomical study of, 167–68 n. 58
    exclusion from medical practice, 17,
        119, 136, 149
    literacy of, 19–21
    and medical schools, xv, 149, 151–52
    oppression of, 150
    as physicians, xv, 148, 151–52
    restriction of roles, 135–36

treatment in courts, 95–96
    vulnerability to witchcraft accusa-
        tions, 44, 111, 131–33, 170 n. 61
    See also Doctoresses; Housewives;
        Midwives; Women healers
Women healers, 96–97, 143
    advocacy by, 88–89, 93–94, 100
    authority of, xii–xiii, 97–98, 103–7,
        111–13
    double role of, 109–10, 112
    enforcement of social norms, 107–9
    gender ambiguity of, 110–11
    gentlewomen, 75–76, 118
    medical notebooks of, 17–19, *18*
    role in paternity suits, 98–100
    See also Davenport, Elizabeth; Doc-
        toresses; Housewives; Hutchinson,
        Ann; Midwives; Physicians; Witch-
        craft trials
Women's communities
    and Ann Hutchinson, 85–89
    and barter economy, 54–55, 161 n. 29
    interaction with men's communities,
        xii, 60–62, 64, 67, 69
    and kin networks, 51–53
    loyalties within, 63–67
    origins of, 45–47
    pursuit of justice by, 68–70
    and witchcraft trials, 55–60
    See also Medical gatherings, women's
Women's movement, 148, 150–51
Wood, Gordon, 83
Woodbridge, Joseph, xii
Wooley, Elizabeth. *See* Davenport, Eliza-
    beth
Woostin, Elizabeth, 64–65

Zanckey (African slave), 120–21